# INSTRUCTOR'S RESOURCE AND METHODS HANDBOOK FOR HEALTH EDUCATION

ALLYN AND BACON, INC.

BOSTON   LONDON   SYDNEY

*PHYLLIS G. ENSOR*
ASSOCIATE PROFESSOR OF HEALTH EDUCATION
TOWSON STATE UNIVERSITY

*RICHARD K. MEANS,*
PROFESSOR AND COORDINATOR OF HEALTH EDUCATION
AUBURN UNIVERSITY

# INSTRUCTOR'S RESOURCE AND METHODS HANDBOOK FOR HEALTH EDUCATION

Second Edition

ISBN 0-205-06750-6

# CONTENTS

# PREFACE ఴ

This *Handbook* has been designed to provide the health instructor with useful suggestions, guidelines, resources, and educational theory. It will also facilitate the
use of *Personal Health: Confronting Your Health Behavior,* by Ensor, Henkel, and
Means (Allyn and Bacon, 1977), and Foundations of Health Science, third edition,
by Henkel, Means, Sawrey and Smolensky (Allyn and Bacon, 1977). Because it was
developed to assist the health instructor to be more than a provider of information,
some of its sections may be useful to others in the health education field.

Teachers and curriculum specialists should find the *Handbook* a valuable resource. Instructors of undergraduate and graduate teacher education courses may
find that the *Handbook* provides a basic framework for giving students an overview
of some of the methods and materials used in health education.

The *Handbook* is compact, and references to more complete sources are included in most sections. We hope health instructors will be motivated to pursue
interests in directions that will add understanding of the learning process in health
education.

Grateful acknowledgment is made to the many students and co-health
educators who have offered suggestions and material for this book. Particular
thanks are due to health education major students who contributed criticism and
enthusiasm for teaching strategies. They are Diane Maloy, Mary Schatz, Mary
Jagerman, and Lynn Rhodes. Health education teachers who helped to pre-test
ideas and materials are Sally Easterbrook and Joan McMahon of Towson State
University.

INSTRUCTOR'S RESOURCE AND METHODS
HANDBOOK FOR HEALTH EDUCATION

# Part One ❦

In this section, an overview of approaches, techniques, and materials available for the professional health educator is provided. Emphasis is placed on those approaches most likely to influence the health behavior of students.

# Chapters ఴ

# WHAT IT'S ALL ABOUT

*Part One ❧ Chapter 1*

The real value of health education lies in its influence on health behavior. That is the final test of health education and represents the basic challenge to the health instructor. It is hoped that learning opportunities provided in the basic health education course will provide a foundational framework for health action in the future life of each student.

This handbook has been prepared to assist health instructors in planning and presenting a dynamic health education course that meets the needs of students today. A health education course can provide students with an opportunity—perhaps the only systematic opportunity—to reflect upon themselves, their development, their needs and their capacities. By the time students reach college, they have a significant set of attitudes about health, but all too often their beliefs are not consistent with behavior. For example, consider the common and sometimes socially condoned habit of smoking. Although students may be fully cognizant of the long-term effects of this habit, they may be apathetic to its protracted consequences.

Thus, health education today is concerned primarily with the behaviors that contribute directly to health. Knowledge and attitude, though important, may not necessarily be causally related to behavior. The health educator then, needs to be concerned with ways of influencing positive changes in health-related behavior—in persuading students to act in ways that will promote optimum health.

Over the years, we have successfully used the ideas presented in this handbook. The behavioral approach has changed student attitude toward required health courses from negative uninvolvement to positive interest and has resulted in behavioral changes. Although full understanding of the dynamics of the factors involved in influencing behavior is yet to come, we feel that this approach is the essence of health education.

The ideas presented in this handbook should aid the instructor who desires to break away from the strict lecture method. A behavioral approach to health education can bring relevancy, personal involvement, and zest into the classroom. Few students fail to respond when material is geared to their needs; when each class period provides an opportunity to become physically, mentally, and, perhaps, emotionally involved. The instructor should be aware that instructional direction may be the fulcrum upon which the desired health behavior of the student turns. If instructors perceive themselves both as individuals and as persons who guide students toward behavioral change, they can quickly establish a warm rapport with their students. The teachers are no longer reservoirs of facts, but persons keenly interested in aiding each student in maximizing full health potential.

Concepts and supporting data can provide the needed background for behavioral change. We suggest approaches and activities, coordinated with reading lists and audiovisual aids, that may assist the instructor in inducing desired behavioral changes. Rather than rigidly following the ideas presented, instructors should implement their own special talents to branch to activities that are more meaningful for an individual class or student. This handbook should help the health educator develop concepts that are most pertinent to healthful living today, as well as suggesting more healthful alternatives to current health behavior.

Any number of class syllabi can be developed. There is never enough class time to learn everything about healthful living. Emphasis should be placed upon the overriding concepts considered appropriate in each particular situation. The suggested student activities, discussion questions, and other aids to instruction set forth in this handbook offer many concrete suggestions for adapting to differing teaching needs.

It is not feasible to propose any detailed suggestions for specific content inclusion. Decisions regarding the sequence and detail of coverage should be reserved for each instructor. However, several sample syllabi are included to provide some assistance in planning.

# PERSONAL PHILOSOPHY OF HEALTH EDUCATION

To be an effective provider of health information, an instructor must know the mechanics of classroom teaching. Equally important, however (and sometimes more important), is the instructor's personal operating philosophy. Health is a way of living, coping with events and environmental hazards. Therefore, health educators as individuals with their own Gestalts must be aware of their personal educational philosophy and their impact as facilitators for more effective (healthful) living.

The personal philosophy and value system that the health educator has about health, life styles, and the nature of the learning process will influence the selection of educational goals, strategies to achieve those goals, and evaluation of progress toward the educational goals of his or her clients. Conscious awareness of their *own* philosophies and roles will provide health teachers with a perspective and a basis for decision making. As health educators are open to attack by other health professionals and the community, this awareness may help keep the educators out of hot water on critical health issues.

"Getting one's head together" is a necessary process for the neophyte as well as the seasoned health educator. Society and social values of illness, health, life, and death are rapidly changing. To be effective, the health educator must be able to define his or her position and ably defend that position, basing the defense on logic and scientific evidence rather than personal opinion alone.

Affirmation and reaffirmation of their personal educational philosophy and theories of health behavior also will help health educators evaluate new theories and teaching methods. It is the unique systematic application of these principles of learning and strategies of teaching that make health education the dynamic and growing profession it is today. As the payoff from classroom activities may be years removed from the present, it is of utmost importance that health education teachers carefully decide for themselves "What It's All About."

## Suggested Readings on Health Philosophy and Theories of Health Behavior

Abijah, Josephine M., "A Philosophy of Health Education," *International Journal of Health Education*, 12:118-120, 1969.

Antonovsky, Aaron, and Harriet Hartman, "Delay in Detection of Cancer: A Review of the Literature," S.O.P.H.E., *Health Education Monographs*, 2:98-128, Summer, 1974.

Allen, Dwight W., "And How They Mangle the Young," *Psychology Today*, 5:71-72, 100, March, 1971.

Becker, Marshall H., "The Health Belief Model and Sick Role Behavior," *S.O.P.H.E. Health Education Monographs*, 2:409-419, Winter, 1974.

"Can Other People's Smoke Hurt You?" *Changing Times*, 29:11-12, September, 1975.

Colley, J., "Passive Smoking in Children," *Nursing Times*, 71:1858-59, 20, November, 1975.

Clarke, Kenneth S., and Guy S. Parcel, "Values and Risk-Taking Behavior: The Concept of Calculated Risk," *Health Education*, 6:26-29, November-December, 1975.

"Education May Not Help," *Medical World News*, 16:7-8, March, 1975.

Haggerty, Robert J., "Changing Lifestyles to Improve Health," *Preventive Medicine*, 6:276-289, 1977.

Harris, William H., "Some Reflections Concerning Approaches to Death Education," *The Journal of School Health*, 48:162-65, March, 1978.

Horine, Field, "Towards a Philosophy of Health Education: Some Preliminary Ideas and Problems," *International Journal of Health Education*, 9:106-112, July-September, 1966.

"Health Belief Model," *S.O.P.H.E. Health Education Monographs*, 2: entire issue, Winter, 1974.

Hochbaum, Godfrey, *Health Behavior: Basic Concepts*, Belmont, Calif.: Wadsworth Publishing Company, 1970.

Kahn, Carol, "Can We Ever Be Really Healthy?" *Family Health*, 10:34-37, 50, January, 1978.

Korscht, John P., "The Health Belief Model and Illness Behavior," *S.O.P.H.E., Health Education Monographs*, 2:387-408, Winter, 1974.

Lawrence, Harry, and Claude L. Walter, "Testing a Behavioral Approach with Group," *Social Work*, 23:127-33, March, 1978.

Oberman, Edna, "Educational Model in Behavioral Training," *Social Work*, 23:120-26, March, 1978.

Restak, Richard, "The Danger of Knowing Too Much," *Psychology Today*, 9: 21, 22, 23, 88, 92, 93, September, 1975.

Rosenstock, Irwin M., "What Research in Motivation Suggests for Public Health," *American Journal of Public Health*, 50:295-302, March, 1960.

Salk, Jonas, "What Do We Mean by Health?" *Health Education*, 9:14-16, January-February, 1978.

Simmonds, Scott, "The Life Span of the Health Educator," *International Journal of Health Education*, 15:3-11, 1972.

Watkin, Donald M., "Personal Responsibility: Key to Effective and Cost Effective Health," *Family and Community Health*, 1:1-7, April, 1978.

Weber, Carol, "A Comparison of Values Clarification and Lecture Methods in Health Education," *The Journal of School Health*, 48:269-73, B.B.

## WRITING BEHAVIORAL OBJECTIVES

Although behavioral objectives are provided at the beginning of each chapter in Part 2 of this *Handbook*, instructors should not adopt those objectives until they have assessed the health education needs of each student and each class as a whole. Additional behavioral objectives may be necessary, and some may be eliminated. The following sources review the basics of writing behavioral objectives:

Cyrs, Thomas E., Jr., *You, Behavioral Objectives and Nutrition Education,* Chicago, Ill.: The National Dairy Council, 1976. (Single copies free from local Dairy Councils.)

Mager, Robert F., *Preparing Instructional Objectives,* Palo Alto, Calif.: Pearon Publishers, 1962.

Walbesser, Henry H., *Constructing Behavioral Objectives,* College Park, Md.: Bureau of Educational Research and Field Studies, College of Education, University of Maryland, 1970.

Each of the above sources was written to teach the preparation of behavioral objectives through a programmed learn-to-do-by-doing method. Upon completing the books, the reader will have gained technical competency to construct educational objectives in behavioral terms.

Those who are not yet convinced of the usefulness of writing behavioral objectives for health teaching might consult "Behavioral Objectives: A Process Approach to Health Education," by Marion B. Pollack, *International Journal of Health Education,* 13:27-35, 1970. Dr. Pollack traces the behavioral objectives movement over the last 30 years. She points out similarities with other educational practices and provides a succinct "Conclusions" section with a perspective for the use of behavior-oriented educational objectives.

A concise debate of the issues related to the use of behavioral objectives is presented by Stephen Isaac and William B. Michael in the *Handbook in Research and Evaluation,* San Diego: Robert R. Knapp, 1972, pp. 162-177.

The following additional materials explaining how to prepare and assess educational goals are available from Insgroup, Inc., 16052 Beach Boulevard, Huntington Beach, California 92647.

Reference Wall Chart—"Objectives for Instructional Programs" $3.00 (multicolored, 19" × 24")

Reference Wall Chart—"Evaluation of Instructional Programs" $3.00 (multicolored, 19" × 24")

## TEACHER-ORIENTED BEHAVIORAL OBJECTIVES FOR HEALTH TEACHING

At the completion of the course the teacher should have done the following:[1]

1. Personally communicated as a human being to other human

[1] An attempt has been made to word these teacher-oriented objectives in realistic, performance, and measurable terms.

beings who have come to him or her during the semester to learn about their health.

2. Made wholehearted attempts to get to know names, faces, and personalities of as many students as possible.

3. Provided health information in a clear, unified, and organized manner through a variety of teaching methods according to sound educational theory.

4. Attended to the attitudes and values of students as they relate to health and systematically helped the students to recognize and evaluate their personal attitudes and values and their contribution to optimal health.

5. Systematically helped students to identify their personal health hazards and to evaluate their health practices in terms of reducing health risks.

6. Informed the students of the grading system and established objective and fair criteria for grading.


## AFFECTIVE EDUCATION
### (Teaching Methods Directed at Clarification of Values Related to Health)

The teaching activities that have come to be categorized as *values clarification teaching* are used in many classrooms to enable students to examine the things that they prize, or value, in relationship to their health. Through these activities, the students make decisions that define their values and how they arrived at their values.

Most teaching methods traditionally used by health teachers have been directed at the cognitive domain. The values clarification activities are directed at the affective domain. According to Rosenstock's Health Belief Model, it is the combination of these two domains that influences and determines health behavior. The writings of a number of educators and psychologists (Raths, Howe, Simons, Harmin, Kirschenbaum, Combs, Stanford, and others) have provided a *systematic* group of activities for the health teacher to use in teaching directed at the affective domain. (It should be cautioned that all affective education [values clarification] has not been thoroughly documented as effective educational practice. Educators, who are sometimes prone to unconditionally accept the latest thing, should study each activity carefully and attend workshops and seminars before using the activities.)

Many questions about value theory in health education remain unanswered. Further research is needed to clarify the worth of values clarification activities in health teaching. The rationale behind their use is that knowledge alone does not change behavior and that, ultimately, individuals are responsible for their own actions and their own health.

Some misunderstandings have arisen concerning the use of "values" teaching activities in the classroom. Each teacher must realize that community boards of education and college deans have differing views on the role and functions of the health teacher. One of the purposes of values clarification activities is to increase the respect that individuals have for others who may hold different opinions. In an increasingly complex democracy, this respect for differences is increasingly needed. As the content of the health education curriculum frequently relates to personal and community values related to health (for example, should the County or City spend limited funds on the school lunch program or repair potholes in the streets?), it seems appropriate to use values clarification activities in the health classroom. However, each practicing health educator must select values strategies that are appropriate for the identified health need, just as he or she must select appropriate cognitive teaching strategies.

In values clarification procedures, the teacher's role is best described as a facilitator: a person who guides, questions, and motivates students to analyze and arrive at their own decisions. Readings related to values clarification teaching may be found in several different branches of the humanistic education movement. Other terms for the teaching techniques include education of self, affective education, achievement motivation training, human development exercises, and open classroom teaching. The following list provides some readings to give the health teacher a basic understanding of affective education activities. Affective education is not recommended as the sole teaching method to be used by the health teacher. It is most effective when balanced with cognitive material. As there is much misinformation and lack of information about health, the presentation of factual material should not be neglected. The decision-making process is based partly on affect and partly on cognition; therefore, both groups of teaching activities are appropriate.

## Suggested Readings on Values Clarification Teaching

Abidin, R.R., Jr., "What's Wrong with Behavior Modification," *Journal of School Psychology*, 9:38-42, 1971.

Combs, Arthur W., Robert A. Blume, Arthur J. Newman, and Hannelore L. Wass, *Professional Education of Teachers*, Boston: Allyn and Bacon, 1974.

Dalis, G. T., and Strasser, *"Teaching Strategies for Values Awareness and Decision Making In Health Education,* New Jersey: Charles B. Slack, Inc., 1977.

Elder, Carl A., *Making Value Judgments: Decisions for Today,* Charles E. Merrill Publishing Co., 1972. (With Teacher's Manual)

Fargo, George A., Charlene Behrns, and Patricia Nolan, *Behavior Modification in the Classroom,* Belmont, Calif.: Wadsworth Publishing Co., 1970.

Greenberg, Jerrol S., "Behavior Modification and Values Clarification and Their Research Implications," *The Journal of School Health,* 55:91-95, February, 1975.

Howe, Leland, and Hart, Gordon, "Counseling with a Focus on Values," *Education,* 97:237-241, Spring, 1977.

Osman, Jack D., and Bonnie Kenny, "Value Growth through Drug Education," *School Health Review,* 25-30, January-February, 1974.

Raths, Louis E., Merrill Harmin, and Sidney B. Simon, *Values and Teaching,* Columbus, Ohio: Charles E. Merrill Publishing Co., 1966.

Read, Donald, and Sidney B. Simon, *Humanistic Education Sourcebook.* Englewood Cliffs, N.J.: Prentice-Hall, 1975.

Reed, D. A., *Looking in: Exploring One's Personal Health Values,* Englewood Cliffs, New Jersey: Prentice-Hall, 1977.

Rees, Floyd D., "Teaching Values through Health Education," *School Health Review,* 1:15-17, February, 1970.

Rich, John M., *Education and Human Values,* Reading, Mass.: Addison-Wesley Publishing Co., 1968.

*School Health Review,* Featured Issue on Values Clarification, Vol. 5, January-February, 1974.

Shostrom, Everett, *Man, the Manipulator,* New York: Bantam Books, 1971.

Simon, Sidney, Leland Howe, and Howard Kirschenbaum, *Values Clarification,* New York: Hart Publishing Co., 1971.

Simon, Sidney; Leland Howe, and Howard Kirschenbaum, *Values Clarification: A Handbook of Practical Strategies for Teachers & Students.* New York: Hart Publishing Co., 1972.

Simon, Sidney, Howard Kirschenbaum, *Readings in Values Clarification.* Minneapolis: Winston Press, 1973.

"Special Feature in Values," *Today's Education,* 66:62-77, January-February 1977.

Stanford, Gene, and Albert E. Roark, *Human Interaction in Education,* Boston: Allyn and Bacon, 1974.

*Values Education in the Public Schools in Hawaii,* Office of Instructional Services, Department of Education, State of Hawaii, January, 1973.

Weinstein, Gerald, and Mario D. Fantini, *Toward Humanistic Education: A Curriculum of Affect,* New York: Praeger Publishers, 1970.

## ASSESSMENT AND EVALUATION IN HEALTH EDUCATION

The words *assessment* and *evaluation* may be new to some health educators. However, they are not new words to other health professionals. In nursing, the "nursing process" is based on the following steps, which are modified from the scientific method: assessment, planning, implementation, and evaluation.[2] The cardinal rule in medicine is that an accurate diagnosis must be made before beginning any treatment regimen, or therapy. Unfortunately, this procedure has not been systematically followed by health educators.

As a professional, the health educator should consider the educational assessment as the first step in preparing the lesson plan or course plan. The purpose is an educational outcome (preferably in behavioral terms), not merely the covering of x amount of material. The use of the educational assessment is teaching oriented toward student health needs, not "covering the material."

The American Hospital Association has prepared an "educational prescription" suitable for educators.[3] The steps in the education prescription are the following: Step I—Identifying the Educational Needs of Patient and Family; Step II—Establishing Educational Goals for Patient and Family; Step III—Select Appropriate Educational Methods; Step IV—Carry out the Educational Program; Step V—Evaluate Patient and Family Education. Although these steps are stated in terms of patient education, the process is the same for any educational plan or setting.

Evaluation of the education activities is carried out in terms of the specific objectives defined in the assessment and goal-setting process. If educational objectives have been stated in realistic, measurable terms, the evaluation methodology may be easily identified. Educational objectives may be written in cognitive, affective, or psychomotor terms. Evaluation then follows the same format. Evaluation by means other than paper-and-pencil tests is en-

2. Helen Yura and Mary B. Walsh, *The Nursing Process: Assessing, Planning, Implementation, Evaluation,* 2nd ed., New York: Appleton-Century-Crofts, 1973.
3. "Strategies for Patient Education," Report of the Second Invitational Conference American Hospital Association, Chicago, 1969, p. 35; *A Model for Planning Patient Education, An Essential Component of Health Care,* Report of the Committee on Educational Tasks in Chronic Illness, Public Health Education Section, American Public Health Association. H.E.W. Publication, HSM, 73-4028.

couraged. Students should be involved both in diagnosing their own health status and in establishing their educational goals. Likewise; participating in evaluation is useful in promoting full involvement and enhancing learning through all the steps in learning.

## Suggested Reading on Assessment and Evaluation

Adkins, Dorothy, *Test Construction: Development and Interpretation of Achievement Tests,* 2nd ed., Columbus, Ohio: C. E. Merrill Publishing Co., 1974.

Burbach, Harold J., and Larry E. Decker, *Plann g and Assessment in Community Education,* Midland, Michigan: Pendell Publishing Company 977.

Good, Cart V., *Essentials of Educational Research,* 2nd ed., New Yor Appleton-Century-Croft, 197 .

Grondland, Norman Edward, *Constructing Achievement Tests,* 2nd ed., Englewood Cliffs, N. J.: Prentice-Hall, 1977.

Means, Richard K., "Research Needs in School Health," *Journal of School Health,* 35:78-85, February, 1965.

Popham, W. James, *Evaluation in Education,* Los Angeles: McCutchan Publishing Corporation, 1974.

Read, Donald A., and Sidney B. Simon, *Humanistic Education Sourcebook,* Englewood Cliffs, N.J.: Prentice-Hall, 1975.

Robinson, R. E., and D. T. Miles, "Behavioral Objectives: An Even Closer Look," *Educational Technology,* 11:39-44, 1971.

Shaw, M. S., and J. C. Wright, *Scales for the Measurement of Attitudes,* New York: McGraw-Hill Book Co., 1967.

Walberg, Herbert, J., *Evaluating Educational Performance,* Berkeley, Calif.: McCutchan Publishing Corporation, 1974.

## Additional Sources

Instructional Objectives Exchange, P.O. Box 24905, Los Angeles, Calif. 90024

General Learning Corporation, 5454 Wisconsin Ave. N.W., Washington, D.C. 20015

Directory of Sources of Measurement Objectives, Dr. John Ahlenius, Consultant, Assessment and Evaluation, State Office Building, Denver, Colo., 80203

# PUTTING IT TOGETHER

*Part One & Chapter 2*

This chapter is composed of a collection of materials to help the health teacher prepare and organize class activities. The Quick Reference Sections and the Health Hazard Appraisals can direct the teacher to sources of up-to-date information and supplementary teaching materials. Regular contact with these organizations will insure prompt delivery of materials and new information as it becomes available.

**COURSE NUMBER:**
**COURSE TITLE:**
**INSTRUCTOR:**
**COURSE OBJECTIVES: The Student**

1. Relates the basic factual information in the various content areas of health science that serves as a basis in helping to meet personal health needs and problems.
2. Interprets the place of health and health education in the broader educational and social perspective.
3. Critically evaluates health information, materials, products, common beliefs, and services in order to establish a sound basis for personal action.
4. States personal health needs and problems, functions effectively within personal limitations, and solves personal health problems by making full use of available resources and services.
5. Cites certain local, state, national, and global health problems and some of the ways in which they might be alleviated.
6. Identifies attitudes and wholesome health behavior that are conducive to maintaining and improving personal and community health.

## BASIC TEXTBOOK AND SUPPLEMENTARY MATERIALS

Henkel, Barbara O., Richard K. Means, James M. Sawrey, and Jack Smolensky,
   *Foundations of Health Science*, 3rd ed., Boston: Allyn and Bacon, 1977.
See bibliography lists for periodical references and supplementary reading suggestions.

## CLASS PARTICIPATION

Attend class regularly, arrive punctually, and clarify all excused absences with the instructor.
Enthusiastically participate in class discussion and other individual and group activities.
Some group work, in addition to individual assignments, may be required.

## QUIZZES, EXAMINATIONS, AND WRITTEN ASSIGNMENTS

Short announced or unannounced quizzes will be given at various times throughout the course.
A mid-term examination may be given, and a final comprehensive examination will be required.
Short written assignments, ordinarily of a research nature, may be given at various times throughout the course.
Written work should be completed on time, properly organized, nearly done, and properly documented.
All written assignments should be typewritten, if possible, and carbon copies should be made.

## OTHER SUGGESTIONS

Final grades will be based upon written reports, quizzes and examinations, individual and group projects, contributions to class discussion, and other work during the course.
Final grades may be determined by a "contract system" whereby the student contracts to perform certain activities to acceptable standards. This contract is negotiated at the beginning of the course.
A variety of methods, techniques, and procedures will be utilized, depending upon the class, to facilitate the learning process and provide a basis for evaluation.
Emphasis throughout the course will be upon current developments in the health sciences and problems of a personal and community health nature.

# EXAMPLE OF DAILY PLANNING FORM

| DAY | DATE | TOPIC | ASSIGNMENTS |
|-----|------|-------|-------------|
|     |      |       |             |
|     |      |       |             |
|     |      |       |             |
|     |      |       |             |
|     |      |       |             |
|     |      |       |             |
|     |      |       |             |
|     |      |       |             |
|     |      |       |             |
|     |      |       |             |
|     |      |       |             |
|     |      |       |             |
|     |      |       |             |
|     |      |       |             |
|     |      |       |             |
|     |      |       |             |
|     |      |       |             |
|     |      |       |             |
|     |      |       |             |
|     |      |       |             |
|     |      |       |             |
|     |      |       |             |
|     |      |       |             |
|     |      |       |             |
|     |      |       |             |
|     |      |       |             |

# SAMPLE PLANNING FORMAT

TITLE

INTRODUCTION

BEHAVIORAL OBJECTIVES

    Knowledge (cognitive)

    Attitudes (affective)

    Practices (action or psychomotor)

INITIATION

DEVELOPMENT

| Content | Estimated Time | Materials | Learning Opportunities |
|---------|----------------|-----------|------------------------|
|         |                |           |                        |

CULMINATION

ANTICIPATED PROBLEMS:

POSSIBLE SOLUTIONS:

EVALUATION

# CONTRACT GRADING SYSTEM

In recent years the contract grading system has gained popularity among students and instructors. The value of the contract system is that it involves the student in setting course and grade objectives. The following is an example of a contract grading system for a general college health course.

## GRADING

Typically, the student enrolling in a course is filled with trepidation concerning the evaluatory procedure. In order to alleviate the traumatic nature of the grading procedure, you are asked to read the following contract. This contract is provided to inform you of the expectations and competencies that are necessary to obtain the letter grade described. After you have arrived at a decision, please record the grade in the space provided at the bottom of the sheet and then affix your signature in the space provided. The grade of NC (no credit) will be issued if a student has not met with his instructor for *at least* one evaluation prior to the last six weeks of the semester. (Exceptions may be considered by instructor.)

## Contract

To attain a C grade, it will be necessary to:

A. Pass all evaluations.

B. Submit three (3) book reviews on topics of your choosing. The only requirement is that they pertain to your health or that of the community.

C. Undertake one activity either as an individual or as part of a group that is aimed at improving your health or that of the community. This involvement may be undertaken once or several times in succession.

To attain a B grade, it will be necessary to:

A. Complete all of the above under the C grade.

B. Undertake a student involvement project that should last approximately ten weeks. The student involvement project is to provide you with the opportunity to engage in some activity that applies directly or indirectly to your health. Choose *either* a self-improvement project *or* a community service project.

To attain an A grade, it will be necessary to:

A. Complete all of the requirements under the C grade.

B. Undertake one of the involvement project options under the B grade.

C. Select a health issue relevant to the seventies that is of special interest to you and then conduct a research project. This research project may be in the form of a library research paper or a critical-issue paper.

Note: All projects and/or ideas can be negotiated; however, all projects must be approved by the instructor in order to be accepted.

I have read and I understand the conditions outlined herein for successful attainment of the grade _____ in this Current Health Problems course.

Date: _____ Signature: _____

## SAMPLE LESSON

### TIME: 40 MINUTES-60 MINUTES

### Introduction

This lesson is a demonstration lesson. The process of behavior change is examined through examples and discussion.

### Concepts and Objectives

Health education today is concerned with action directly contributing to health. The purpose of this lesson, in addition to knowledge and attitude change, is to lead students to act in ways that will promote optimum health. During the lesson, the class should together seek to:

1. Identify several smokers who may have habits that will seriously endanger their health.

2. Persuade the smokers to stop smoking or cut down appreciably.

3. Identify nonsmokers and determine their propensity to begin smoking or remain nonsmokers.

4. Identify former smokers, determine their motivation and method of quitting, and have them share their experience with others.

---

## Discussion and Group Procedures

### INTRODUCTION TO THE PROBLEM

Through a show of hands, find several students in the class who smoke cigarettes. Ask for two or three to come to the front of the class with the instructor. Ask the volunteers to identify themselves and tell a few things about themselves (for example, home town, major interests). Try to have the students relax, if possible.

### EXPLORATION

Ask each student the following questions (or others if more appropriate) to explore smoking habits. Depending on the direction of the discussion, it may be appropriate to thoroughly question one student at a time or to ask all students the same question before going on to the next question. (1) Do you smoke cigarettes? What kind? (2) How long have you been smoking? (3) What kind of a habit do you have now? (4) How much money do you spend daily, weekly, for cigarettes? (5) Who made you start smoking? (Answer will most probably be "No one made me start to smoke.") (6) Well, why did you start to smoke? (Explore: rephrase and ask if you understand the reasons correctly.) (7) Is that the reason why you smoke now? Why do you continue to smoke? (8) Do you know the dangers of smoking? (9) Why do you continue to smoke even though you know the dangers of smoking? (10) Have you ever wanted to, or tried to, stop smoking? Tell us about it. (Explore success or failure.)

Direct the following questions to the class. (1) What do you think of this student's smoking habit? (2) Is this person being honest? (3) Has this person really tried to stop? (4) Why do you think there was success or failure in the efforts to stop? (Follow the same line of questioning and reacting with other student smokers.)

### ACTION OR DECISION

After the discussion, have the volunteers discuss what they now think about their smoking habits. Follow with questions directed at what their future behavior may be. If they desire to stop smoking, find out how they plan to go about it. Discuss this. Ask the class if they think any of the volunteers will be successful. Explore to seek solutions, focusing attention on the volunteers. Turn the discussion, then, to include any other students in the class who smoke and may wish help in stopping.

## REVIEW AND CONCLUSIONS

Review the concept that knowledge and attitude alone do not necessarily change behavior—emotions, feelings, and habits also must be considered. Follow with free discussion on behavior and habits. Ask the class what can motivate a person to change personal health habits. In other words, what motivates people to adopt good health habits, or change habits, since knowledge alone seems to motivate few people? Explore the effect of fear and other factors.

NOTE: A change in these students' smoking habits may not be effected. Indeed, they may not even want to stop smoking, or they may want to smoke more since they were nervous in front of the class. The process is the important thing in this lesson. The nature of, and problems in, current health education will have been demonstrated on a personal level.

## Student Readings

"Can Other People's Smoke Hurt You?" *Changing Times*, 29:11-12, September, 1975.

Colley, John, "Passive Smoking in Children," *Nursing Times*, 71: 1858-59, November 20, 1975.

Doyle, Nancy C., "The Facts about Second-hand Cigarette Smoke," *American Lung Association Bulletin*, 60:13-15, July, 1974.

Jones, Philippa, "Smoking and Pregnancy," *Nursing Times*, 71:2038-39, December 18, 1975.

Olshavsky, R. W., *No More Butts: A Psychologist's Approach to Quitting Cigarettes*, Bloomington, Indiana: Indiana University Press, 1977.

Mauer, H., and J. Schwartz, "Do Smokers' Clinics Really Work?" *Science Digest*, 78:72-76, September, 1975.

Meredity, H.V., "Relationship between Tobacco Smoking of Pregnant Women and Body Size of Offspring," *Human Biology*, 47:451-72, December, 1975.

"No Smoking—Some States Mean It," *U.S. News and World Report*, 79:45, October 20, 1975.

Pederson, L.L., et al., "Comparison of Hypnosis plus Counseling, Counseling Alone, and Hypnosis Alone in a Community Service Smoking Withdrawal Program," *Journal of Consulting and Clinical Psychology*, 43:920, December, 1975.

"Social Smoking," *Science Digest*, 79:24, January, 1976.

*The Dangers of Smoking — The Benefits of Quitting*, New York: The American Cancer Society, 1972.

"Want to Quit Smoking? Here Are Tested Ways," *Today's Health*, 47:84-86, May, 1969.

# QUICK REFERENCE:  AGENCIES INVOLVED
# IN HEALTH AND HEALTH EDUCATION

*(For easy reference, write in the names and addresses of your state and local organizations)*

## OFFICIAL AGENCIES

State Health Department _____

_____

Phone: _____

Local _____

_____

Phone: _____

State Department of Education _____

_____

Phone: _____

County or Local _____

_____

Phone: _____

## PROFESSIONAL AGENCIES

State Health Association _____

_____

Phone: _____

Other Organizations _____

_____

Phone: _____

_____

_____

Phone: _____

# QUICK REFERENCE: PERIODICAL SOURCES
# OF HEALTH INFORMATION

*American Heart Journal*, monthly, 3207 Washington Boulevard, St. Louis, Mo. 63103.

*American Journal of Nursing*, monthly, 10 Columbus Circle, New York, N.Y. 10019.

*American Journal of Public Health*, monthly, American Public Health Association, 1015 Eighteenth Street, N. W., Washington, D. C. 20036.

*Children*, bi-monthly, Office of Child Development, U.S. Department of Health, Education and Welfare, Washington, D.C. 20402.

*Chronicle of the World Health Organization*, bi-monthly, World Health Organization, Geneva, Switzerland.

*Consumer Reports*, monthly, Consumers Union, Inc., 256 Washington, Mt. Vernon, N.Y. 10850.

*Consumer's Bulletin*, monthly, Consumer's Research, Inc., Washington, N.J. 07882.

*Environment*, 438 N. Skinker Boulevard, St. Louis, Mo. 63130.

*Family Health*, monthly, Family Media, Inc., 149 Fifth Avenue, New York, N. Y. (Incorporates *Today's Health*)

*Futurist*, monthly, World Future Society, P. O. Box 19285, Twentieth Street Station, Washington, D.C. 20036.

*Health Education*, monthly, Association for the Advancement of Health Education, 1201 16th St. N.W., Washington, D.C. 20036.

*International Journal of Health Education*, monthly, International Union for Health Education of the Public, 3 rue Viollier, Geneva, Switzerland.

*Journal of American College Health Association*, formerly *Student Medicine*, quarterly, American College Health Association, Gannett Medical Clinic, Ithaca, N.Y. 14850.

*Journal of American Medical Association*, weekly, American Medical Association, 535 North Dearborn Street, Chicago, Ill. 60610.

*Journal of Marriage and the Family*, 1219 University Avenue, S.E., Minneapolis, Minn. 55414.

*Journal of School Health*, monthly, American School Health Association, 515 East Main Street, Kent, Ohio 44240.

*Mental Health Digest*, monthly, National Institute of Mental Health, Superintendent of Documents, Government Printing Office, Washington, D.C. 20402.

*Mental Hygiene*, quarterly, National Association for Mental Health, 10 Columbus Circle, New York, N.Y. 10019.

*Monthly Vital Statistics Reports*, monthly, U.S. Department of Health, Education, and Welfare, Office of Vital Statistics, Washington, D.C., 20402.

*National Safety News*, monthly, National Safety Council, 425 North Michigan Avenue, Chicago, Ill. 60611.

*Psychology Today*, monthly, Psychology Today, P. O. Box 60407, Terminal Annex, Los Angeles, Calif. 90021.

*PTA Magazine*, monthly, National Congress of Parents and Teachers, 700 North Rush Street, Chicago, Ill. 60611.

*Research Quarterly,* quarterly, American Alliance for Health, Physical Education and Recreation, 1201 Sixteenth Street, N.W., Washington, D.C. 20036.

*Safety,* bi-monthly, National Commission on Safety Education, National Education Association, 1201 Sixteenth Street, N.W., Washington, D.C., 20036.

*Science Digest,* monthly, Science Digest, Inc., 200 East Ontario Street, Chicago, Ill, 60011.

*Statistical Bulletin,* monthly, Metropolitan Life Insurance Company, 1 Madison Avenue, New York, N.Y. 10010.

*World Health,* monthly, World Health Organization, Regional Office for the Americas, Pan American Sanitary Bureau, 1501 New Hampshire Avenue, N.W., Washington, D.C. 20036.

# QUICK REFERENCE MEDICAL TERMS: PREFIXES, SUFFIXES, AND COMBINING TERMS

Health Education instructors and students can understand some of the terminology used in medicine and the health-related sciences by recognizing the meaning of certain parts of words. For example:

| *Prefix* | *Stem* | *Suffix* | *WORD* |
|---|---|---|---|
| ENDO- (within) | CARDI (heart) | -ITIS (inflammation) | ENDOCARDITIS (Inflammation of the endo-cardium or lining of the heart) |

The following list of prefixes, suffixes, and combining forms may be helpful in understanding certain technical terms. Each term is followed by its meaning and a sample word.

## PREFIXES

ad- (near), adrenal
ab- (away from), abnormal
an- (without), anoxia
anti- (against), antibiotic
bio- (life), biology
calor- (heat), calorie

co- (together), coordination
dis- (negative, ill), disease
dys- (difficult), dysmenorrhea
endo- (within), endoderm
ex- (out from), exhale
hemo- (blood), hemorrhage

hyper- (excessive), hypertension
hypo- (under), hypoglycemia
im- (in), impacted
macro- (large), macrocyte
micro- (small), microscope

peri- (around), periodontal
post- (after), postmortem
pre- (before), prenatal
re- (again), recurrence
uni- (one), unicellular

## SUFFIXES

-algia (pain), neuralgia
-cide (kill), pesticide
-cule (small), molecule
-ectomy (cut), appendectomy
-emia (blood), anemia
-gram (writing), electrocardiogram
-itis (inflammation), bronchitis

-logy (study of), dermatology
-oid (like), lymphoid
-oma (swelling), carcinoma
-opia (vision), hyperopia
-osis (condition), nephrosis
-rhea (discharge), diarrhea
-therapy (treatment), radiotherapy

## COMMON COMBINING TERMS

arthr (joint), arthritis
cardi (heart), cardiovascular
costo (rib), intercostal
cyta (cell), lymphocyte
denti (tooth), dentition
derm (skin), dermatology
gastr (stomach), gastric
gyn (woman), gynecology
hepat (liver), hepatitis
leuko (white), leukocyte
myo (muscle), myocardium
neo (new), neoplasm

nephro (kidney), nephritis
neur (nerve), neuritis
osteo (bone), osteoarthritis
oto (ear), otitis
path (disease), pathology
phago (to eat), phagocytosis
pod (foot), podiatrist
proto (first), protozoa
psych (mind), psychiatry
pulmo (lung), pulmonary
thermo (heat), thermometer
vaso (vessel), vascular

## QUICK REFERENCE: SOURCES OF GENERAL HEALTH EDUCATION MATERIALS

The following references include descriptive and / or indexed sources of materials. Where to order materials, how to order, cost, and other information relative to the use of certain materials is provided in most of the listings.

Anderson, C. L., *School Health Practice*, 5th ed., St. Louis: C. V. Mosby Co., 1972, pp. 397-424.

Beyrer, Mary K., Ann E. Nolte, and Marian K. Solleder, *A Directory of*

*Selected References and Resources for Health Instruction*, 2nd ed., Minneapolis: Burgess Publishing Co., 1967, 210 pp.

Bedworth, David A., and Albert E. Bedworth, *Health Education: A Process for Human Effectiveness,* New York: Harper & Row, 1978.

Bruess, Clint E., and John E. Gay, *Implementing Comprehensive School Health,* New York: Macmillan, 1978.

Engs, Ruth C., S. Eugene Barnes, and Molly Wantz, *Health Games Students Play,* Dubuque, Iowa: Kendall/Hunt Publishing Company, 1975.

Fodor, John T., and Gus T. Dalis, *Health Instruction: Theory and Application,* Philadelphia: Lea and Febiger, 1966, pp. 157-65.

Foster, Julia C., *The Teaching of Health Education,* Columbus, Ohio: Charles E. Merrill Publishing Co., 1968, pp. 236-61.

Greenberg, Jerrold S., *Student-Centered Health Instruction: A Humanistic Approach,* Reading, Mass.: Addison-Wesley, 1978.

Kilander, H. Frederick, *School Health Education,* 2nd. ed., New York: The Macmillan Co., 1968, pp. 495-509.

Kime, Robert E., Richard Schlaadt, and Lenord Tritsch, *Health Instruction: An Action Approach,* Englewood Cliffs, New Jersey: Prentice-Hall, 1977.

Lemcke, John, and John DeMillion, *278 Experimental Strategies for Instructors of Health,* Dubuque, Iowa: Kendall/Hunt Publishing Company, 1975.

Mayshark, Cyrus, and Leslie W. Irwin, *Health Education in Secondary Schools,* 2nd ed., St. Louis: C. V. Mosby Co., 1968, pp. 261-70.

Nemir, Alma, *The School Health Program,* 3rd ed., Philadelphia: W. B. Saunders Co., 1970, pp. 411-18.

Read, Donald A., and Walter H. Greene, *Creative Teaching in Health,* New York: The Macmillan Co., 1971, pp. 391-419.

Schneider, Robert E., *Methods and Materials of Health Education,* 2nd ed., Philadelphia: W. B. Saunders, 1964, pp. 254-59.

Turner, C. E., Harriet B. Randall, and Sara Louise Smith, *School Health and Health Education,* 6th ed., St. Louis: C. V. Mosby Co., 1970, pp. 239-55.

Annotated Bibliography of Health Games" prepared by Kenneth L. Packer, Regional Health Coordinator, Bureau of Cooperative Education, Yorktown Heights, New York 10598. *The Journal of School Health,* Vol 45, No. 2, pp. 113-116. Packer describes teaching games and comments on their use in the health education class. A good source. Topics of Games: Physical Health, Nutrition, Alcohol, Drugs, Tobacco, Mental Health, and First Aid in Survival.

## QUICK REFERENCE
## MULTI-MEDIA MATERIALS

The following list of audiovisual sources represents the majority of the producers and distributors of health education films and filmstrips. Films available from this listing are described in the individual chapters in Part 2. The teacher should preview each film before use to determine its appropriateness for the desired educational goals. A film or filmstrip can be a powerful educational tool if used correctly. It is suggested that teachers select films that are directed to affective (conscious and subliminal) learning as well as cognitive learning.

Too often in the past, health instructors have used films, filmstrips and other audiovisual materials mainly to provide information. To adequately cover a topic, a film was necessarily twenty minutes to an hour long. Some were excellent on all counts. However, scientific and health advances come so rapidly, films quickly become outdated. Also, lengthy films have become limited in value as instructors have changed the purpose of film use. Multi-Media Materials are now more widely used to introduce a topic, to stimulate discussion and the exchange of ideas, or to review concepts. Most good films for this purpose are limited to 5—15 minutes.

## Sources of Health Films, Filmstrips, and Other Media Teaching Aids

Appropriate and well-selected films and filmstrips are valuable supplementary materials for effective college health instruction. The college or university library, local or state public health department, local or regional voluntary health agencies, and local public library are normally good sources. In addition, the following more specific distributors of films and filmstrips can be helpful:

American Educational Films, 331 North Maple Drive, Beverly Hills, Calif. 90210.

American Film Producers, 1540 Broadway, New York, N.Y. 10036.

American Medical Association, 535 North Dearborn Street, Chicago, Ill. 60610.

Association Films, Inc., 600 Grand Avenue, Ridgefield, N.J. 07657.

Bray Studios, 630 Ninth Avenue, New York, N.Y. 10036.

Churchill Films, 662 N. Robertson Boulevard, Los Angeles, Calif. 90069.

Communications Materials Center, Columbia University Press, Broadway and 11th Avenue, New York, N.Y. 10027.

Contemporary Films, 34 Macquesten Parkway South, Mount Vernon, N.Y. 10550.

Coronet Instructional Films, 65 East South Water Street, Chicago, Ill. 60601.

CRM Educational Films, Del Mar, Calif. 92014. (9263 West 3rd Street, Beverly Hills, Calif. 90210)

Current Affairs, 24 Danbury Road, Wilton, Conn. 06897.

Dynamic Films, Inc., 608 Madison Avenue, New York, N.Y. 10022.

Educators Guide to Free Films, Educators Progress Service, Randolph, Wis. 53956.

Educators Information Service (free catalog), Bureau of Education and Research, American Advertising Federation, 655 Madison Avenue, New York, N.Y. 10021.

Educators Progress Service, Inc., Randolph, Wis. 53956.

Encyclopedia Britannica Films, Inc., 1150 Wilmette Avenue, Wilmette, Ill. 60091.

Film Distributors International, 1450 Thousand Oaks Boulevard, Thousand Oaks, Calif. 91360.

Guide to Government Loan Film, Serina Press, 70 Kennedy Street, Alexandria, Va. 22305.

Indiana University Audio Visual Center, Bloomington, Ind. 47401.

International Film Bureau, Inc., 332 South Michigan Avenue, Chicago, Ill. 60604.

Lee Creative Communications, Inc., P. O. Box 1367, Rochester, N.Y. 14603.

McGraw-Hill Book Company, Inc., Text-Film Department, 330 West 42nd Street, New York, N.Y. 10036.

Modern Talking Picture Service, Inc., 3 East 54th Street, New York, N.Y. 10022.

Multimedia Fair, Inc., 380 Maple Ave. West, Vienna, Va. 22106.

National Dairy Council, 111 North Canal Street, Chicago, Ill. 60606.

National Medical Audiovisual Center (Annex), Station K, Atlanta, Ga. 30334.

NET Film Service, c/o Audio-Visual Center, Indiana University, Bloomington, Ind. 47401.

Perennial Education, Inc., P.O. Box 236, 1825 Willow Road, Northfield, Ill. 60093.

Popular Science Audio-Visuals, Inc. Times Mirror, 5235 Ravenswood Avenue, Chicago, Ill. 60604.

Sam Orleans Film Productions, 211 Cumberland Avenue, Knoxville, Ind. 37920.

Shell Film Library, 450 North Meridian Street, Indianapolis, Ind. 46204.

Sierra Club, 1050 Mills Tower, 220 Bush Street, San Francisco, Calif. 94104.

Social Science Films, 2710 Hampton Avenue, St. Louis, Mo. 63139.

United States Public Health Service, U.S. Department of Health, Education and Welfare, Washington, D.C. 20025.

United World Films, 221 Park Avenue South, New York, N. Y. 10003.

Visual Teaching Materials (free catalog), Visual Products Division, 3M Company, Box 3344, St. Paul, Minn. 55101.

Young America Films, McGraw-Hill Distributors, Department 423, 1221 Avenue of the Americas, New York, N.Y. 10020.

## SOURCES OF PERSONAL HEALTH HAZARD (RISK) APPRAISAL FORMS

Personal health appraisals (inventories) are teaching aids that can assist the health teacher in personalizing the health course. Unfortunately, many health teachers assume that all college students are equally informed or uninformed about health matters. Quite the contrary. Each student enters the health education class with his or her own medical history and backlog of experiences, attitudes, and knowledges.

Not all checklists, scales and rating forms that have been

published are valid and reliable. However, many are useful in the classroom and can serve as a guide for personal health appraisal and motivation.

> *CAUTION: These paper-and-pencil tests should be used by the classroom teacher in an appropriate manner. They are not guaranteed medical histories or predictors of physical or emotional health, nor are they designed to invade a student's private life. It is suggested that this be explained in the directions before the inventories are utilized in teaching.*

### 1. GENERAL HEALTH STATUS AND KNOWLEDGE—Health Hazard Appraisal

Perhaps the most comprehensive and proven personal health appraisal is the Health Hazard Appraisal developed as a health education tool by Dr. Lewis C. Robbins and associates at the Methodist Hospital of Indiana in Indianapolis.

Health hazards are divided into two categories: those over which the individual has no control (such as heredity) and those over which the individual has control (such as weight, smoking, occupational hazards, and miles driven per year). Life expectancy is computed based on the weighted values of various health hazards each individual has. Accordingly, by reducing health risks over which the individual has control (smoking, tension, weight) the individual can increase his or her computed life expectancy. The individual is questioned regarding his or her values, life style, and health habits and is challenged to reduce health risks.

The Health Hazard Appraisal is a five-page medical history and health practices questionnaire prepared on computer answer sheets. A computer program has been written for quick scoring of large numbers of appraisals. A print-out is provided for each participant with computed life expectancy and instructions regarding how computed life expectancy may be increased by reducing specific health hazards the individual has reported. This appraisal may be obtained from Health Hazard Appraisal, c/o Methodist Hospital of Indiana, 1604 N. Capitol St., Indianapolis, Ind., 46202.

### 2. A BRIEF FORM—Health Hazard Appraisal

A brief form of the Health Hazard Appraisal without personalized computer evaluation may be found in the popular magazine *Family Circle*.

Sehnert, Keith W., and Howard Wisenberg, "Your Real Age Vs. Your Medical Age," *Family Circle*, 86:84-85, August, 1975.

The Health Hazard Appraisal is based on U.S. health statistics and designed to predict a person's probable life expectancy according to selected variables. Some of the variables, such as hereditary factors or sex or chronological age, are not amenable to change; however, other factors, such as smoking or weight control, may indicate that the individual might live longer if he changed his health habits.

### 3. PREVENTIVE MEDICINE GUIDE—
### Risk Factor Questionnaire for Women

Ellen Switzer, "Preventive Medicine Guide—How to Be Healthy at Any Age," *Family Circle*, 86:137-144, April, 1975.

This specially designed health hazard identification list for women was prepared from the Health Hazard Appraisal of the Life Extension Institute of New York City. The form contains twenty-one questions with interpretation of the risks of yes replies to each question. A copy of the questionnaire appears in the *Family Circle* article.

### 4. GENERAL HEALTH KNOWLEDGE

"How Much do You Know About Health?" *Family Health*, 9:60, 61, 64, August, 1975.

This twenty-five-item questionnaire in a multiple-choice format is based on the findings of a survey conducted by Louis Harris for Blue Cross. That survey indicated that although the general public thinks it is well informed about health, in reality it is not.

This questionnaire covers topics such as first aid for shock, common digestive ailments, signs and symptoms of heart attack, leading causes of death in the United States, exercise, nutrition, drugs, sleep, normal delivery of a baby, and warning signs of cancer.

Although this knowledge inventory has not been tested for validity and reliability, it does appear to be a valid mini-quiz to assess general level of health knowledge. Scoring, rating, and instructions for additional health education are provided in the journal article.

## 5. ATTITUDES TOWARD DEATH

Hardt, Dale V., "Development of an Investigatory Instrument to Measure Attitudes toward Death," *The Journal of School Health*, 45:96-99, February, 1975. School of Health Sciences and Physical Education, East Stroudsburg State College, East Stroudsburg, Pennsylvania.

This brief, twenty-item attitude scale attempts to assess the student's attitudes toward death. Reliability estimates indicate a reliability coefficient of .87 (Spearman Brown "Prophecy Formula"). The scale may be used as a pre and post study assessment instrument. There are no right or wrong answers, and the instrument makes no attempt to change a student's attitude or indicate a desired change, or direction of change, of attitude.

A more comprehensive inventory appeared in the August, 1970, issue of *Psychology Today*. This inventory was developed by Edwin Schneidman of the Center for Advanced Study in the Behavioral Sciences with Edwin Parker and G. Ray Funkhouser of Stanford University. It is a revision of an earlier inventory developed by Shneidman when at Harvard University.

The inventory appeared to poll the readers of *Psychology Today*. Over 30,000 questionnaires were returned. Reliability estimates are not given, nor other criteria, however the results that appeared in the June, 1971, issue of *Psychology Today*, explains the limitations.

Permission may be obtained to use this inventory for teaching purposes from Communications Research Machines, Inc., 9263 West 3rd Street, Beverly Hills, California, 90210. Explanation on how the inventory may be used in a teaching unit is given in Joan D. McMahon, "A Unit for Independent Study in Death Education," *School Health Review*, 4:27-34, July-August, 1973.

A comprehensive review of activities and programs of death education has been compiled by the ERIC Clearinghouse on Teacher Education. Write ERIC Clearinghouse on Teacher Education, Suite 616, One Dupont Circle, Washington, D.C. 20036. The booklet is titled *Death Education as a Learning Experience*, 1975.

## 6. DEPRESSION

Cherry, Rona, and Laurence Cherry, "Depression," *Glamour*, 71:202, 203, 220, 228, 232, 234, May, 1974. (From Aaron T. Beck, *Diagnosis and Management of Depression*, New York: University of Pennsylvania Press, 1973.)

This article clearly defines depression as a clinical condition. Signs and symptoms are presented in everyday terms so that the non-clinical reader may identify the signs of clinical depression compared to life's "normal ups and downs." Attention is given to the subtle ways that depression can incapacitate a person and how the individual and his friends and/or family try to deny that the person has a serious problem. The Beck Depression Inventory is reproduced in the article.

**7. STRESS AND EMOTIONAL**
**RESPONSE TO LIFE-EVENTS**
**"What To Do When You're**
**Under Stress"**

U.S. *News & World Report*, 75: 48, 52, 54, September 24, 1973.

This article reviews the life-events scale developed by Dr. Thomas H. Holmes at the University of Washington School of Medicine in Seattle. Dr. Beck has indicated that there is a "reasonably good correlation" between an accumulation of a number of life changes and depression and/or physical illness. Dr. Holmes's study indicates that it may be possible to predict the effects of "future shock" and the rapid rate of life change in physical illness proneness.

The Holmes Life-Events Scale includes items such as divorce, business readjustment, trouble with in-laws, change in work hours, amount of mortgage, retirement, and many other items with designated "impact points." Holmes's study indicates that the accumulation of 200 or more of the "impact points" in a given year may make an individual vulnerable to illness.

An example of the checklist appears in the *U.S. News & World Report* article.

**8. ALCOHOLISM**

Martin, Paul, "Teenage Alcoholism," *Consumers Digest*, 14:20-22. July-August, 1975.

A twenty-question self-quiz similar to the "Twenty Questions" prepared by Alcoholics Anonymous is presented in this article. The article indicates that the questionnaire, developed by Johns Hopkins University in Baltimore, Md., is used in assessing an alcoholic patient.

Similar self-administered quizzes may be obtained from

your local chapters of Alcoholics Anonymous. Each is coded to indicate the degree of a drinking problem or alcoholism according to numbers of "yes" responses.

### 9. SMOKING

The Smoker's Self-Testing Kit was developed by Daniel Horn, Director of the National Clearinghouse for Smoking and Health. The test, in booklet form, may be obtained for ten cents from the Superintendent of Documents, U.S. Government Printing Office, Washington, D.C. 20402. The booklet consists of four short tests to help the individual make his own assessment of his knowledge of cigarette smoking and health and how he feels about smoking. Directions are given for scoring the tests and for interpretation.

A short form designed as a Teen-Age Self-Test is also available. DHEW Publ. No. (CDC) 74-8723, National Clearinghouse for Smoking and Health, Bethesda, Md. 20016.

### 10. PUBLISHED APPRAISALS OF HEALTH ATTITUDES AND HEALTH BEHAVIOR

a. A collection of scales and indices that may be useful to the classroom health educator is compiled in the *Handbook of Scales and Indices of Health Behavior*, by Reeder, Ramacher, and Gorelnik, Pacific Palisades, Calif.: Goodyear Publishing Co., Inc., 1976.

This collection of scales and the descriptions of recent research and projects using these measurement devices are presented in outline format. Samples of the instruments are given as appropriate. This resource should prove valuable to teachers who desire to identify attitudes and behaviors related to health and utilization of health services.

b. One of the most complete collections of instruments is *Measures of Social Psychological Attitudes*, edited by Robinson and Shaver, Ann Arbor, Mich.: Institute for Social Research, University of Michigan, 1973. This volume has been designed for researchers; however, the classroom teacher may find certain instruments useful for teaching purposes. Again, caution should be used with instruments that attempt to measure attitudes. Regulations and policies differ in states and school districts.

c. *Personal Health Appraisal*, Walter D. Sorochan, New York: John Wiley & Sons, 1976.

This handbook is a collection of self-inventories on a wide variety of health topics and module techniques to motivate the individual to alter his or her health behavior. Most of the instruments will spark an interest among students because of the personalized approach. Very few reliability estimates are given for the instruments; however, because of the nature of the instruments, reliability estimates may not be necessary.

## 11. THE SEMANTIC DIFFERENTIAL

The Semantic Differential, devised by Osgood, is a means of measuring the connotative meanings of concepts as points in what is called "semantic space."[1] Osgood explains the basis for measuring concepts by the use of the adjective pairs that compose a semantic differential scale. Characteristics are communicated by adjectives. Therefore, meaning can be measured by measuring the degree of the descriptive adjectives attributed to a concept.

A semantic differential is constructed using adjective pairs that are categorized as representing one of three main dimensions: evaluative, potency, and activity. Osgood has prepared a list of adjective pairs that have been demonstrated to be most useful in measuring the "semantic space."[2]

A semantic differential scale may be analyzed by several different methods: individual profiles may be prepared, group profile means may be compared (e.g., male vs. female scores and parent vs. child scores), and group means on various concepts may be compared (e.g., comparing the concepts *Heart Attack* and *Cancer*). Also, semantic differential scores may be used as pre and post measures.

**Examples of Use of the Semantic Differential in Health Education**

1. Herrick, Jean S., "Dimensions in the Judgement of Illness," *Genetic Psychology Monographs,* 79:191-209, May, 1969.

2. Herrick, Jean S., "The Use of the Semantic Differential: Its Special Application to Illness," *Health Education Monographs,* 29:37-49, 1969.

3. Herrick, Jean S., and Alice M. Heath, "Mexican-American Teenagers' Judgement of Illness: A Case Study of the Use of the Semantic Differential," *Health Education Monographs,* 29:51-58, 1969.

4. Jenkins, C. David, "The Semantic Differential for Health, A Technique for Measuring Beliefs about Disease," *Public Health Reports,* 81:549-58, June, 1966.

1.  Charles Osgood, George J. Suci, and Percy H. Tannenbaum, *The Measurement of Meaning,* Urbana: University of Illinois Press, 1975, p. 4.
2.  *Ibid.,* p. 37.

**Directions:** Place an X mark at the place along each line which represents how you feel the characteristic best describes the word at the top. For example, if you think cancer is contagious, place your X mark as close to the word *contagious* as you can. If you think it is not contagious, place your mark at the opposite end of the line. If you don't know, or are not sure, place your mark in the center of the line.

---

## CANCER

| | | | | | | | |
|---|---|---|---|---|---|---|---|
| Beautiful | 7 | 6 | 5 | 4 | 3 | 2 | 1 : Ugly |
| Soft | 1 | 2 | 3 | 4 | 5 | 6 | 7 : Hard |
| Strong | 1 | 2 | 3 | 4 | 5 | 6 | 7 : Weak |
| Clean | 7 | 6 | 5 | 4 | 3 | 2 | 1 : Dirty |
| Bad | 1 | 2 | 3 | 4 | 5 | 6 | 7 : Good |
| Sharp | 1 | 2 | 3 | 4 | 5 | 6 | 7 : Dull |
| Contagious | 1 | 2 | 3 | 4 | 5 | 6 | 7 : Not Contagious |
| Good | 7 | 6 | 5 | 4 | 3 | 2 | 1 : Bad |
| Sinful | 1 | 2 | 3 | 4 | 5 | 6 | 7 : Pure |

SAMPLE

---

**Scoring:** (Numbers not to be included on form for participant until after form has been completed)

Assign numbers to adjective pairs with low numbers representing the negative and higher numbers representing the positive. (Scale from 1 to 7)

The total of all the scales represents the individual's total score. A profile may be prepared by drawing a line from scale to scale for each participant.

# GETTING IT ACROSS

*Part One* ↗ *Chapter 3*

## THE ART OF TEACHING[1]

There is obviously much more to good teaching than constructing attractive visual materials, running complicated instructional equipment, or organizing and conducting group activities. Effective teaching requires a deep understanding of human nature, individual behavior, group interaction, and the phenomenon of learning itself.

### Values of Meaningful Experience

It is becoming increasingly apparent that concepts and ideas are more easily and firmly grasped when presented in more than one way. Instruction that supplements verbalization with something projected on a screen, drawn on the chalkboard, or resolved through group deliberation is often infinitely more effective.

It is evident that each technique and procedure of instruction has its own characteristics as well as its own unique, fundamental advantages and limitations. The effective use of different teaching methods requires skill in planning, selecting, preparing, adapting, utilizing, and appraising. It also involves a functional understanding of *why* as well as *what* and *how*.

### Basic Classroom Considerations

Certain classroom factors or considerations help stimulate learning.

1. Adapted from Richard K. Means, *Methodology in Education*, Columbus Ohio: Charles E. Merrill, Publishers, 1968, pp. 6-10, copyright 1968; and Stanley Rosenberg and Phyllis G. Ensor, "Learning, Patient Education and Hypertension," in Ivan Borofsky, Ed., *Medication Compliance: A Behavioral Management Approach*, Thorofare, N.J.: Charles B. Slack, Inc., copyright 1977.

Some of these are presented in the following questions, all with strong application to method:

Are assignments clear and specific so that each student knows what is expected?

Are individual differences provided for in the classroom or laboratory setting?

Is the subject matter related to actual life experiences?

Is the worth of each individual recognized, and is creativity rather than conformity encouraged?

Is good use made of all available teaching materials?

Are students evaluated frequently?

Are lines of communication open?

It is clearly evident that teachers guide students by the words they utter, the things they do, the way they act, and the way they manipulate the environment. They influence behavior by providing activities that stimulate student thinking, feeling, and action. They plan experiences that encourage creativity, enriched interests, and originality of expression. They help students to analyze situations, identify their problems, plan and evaluate their progress, and establish worthwhile goals.

## THE LEARNING PROCESS

Much has been written concerning the complex phenomenon of learning. Numerous articles and books have been devoted to an analysis of the factors that influence learning and the elaboration of process by which learning seems most likely to be enhanced. The following material is an attempt to review basic principles of learning.

### Methodology and Learning

Learning has been defined as a consistent change in behavior which, in educational institutions, is brought about by the activities and experiences that are provided by the school. Keeton, in a publication of the Association for Higher Education, realistically proposed that "Courses define only part of the climate of learning, perhaps a minor part." With respect to instructional method, he suggested that "preoccupation with methods of teaching, unless informed by a comprehensive theory about the climate of learning within which they are applied, may prove to be a wasted effort."[2]

Thus, it should be emphasized that teaching methods, procedures, and techniques are not an end in themselves, but are rather a means by which students can be assisted to solve their individual and social problems. They involve the planning and arrangement of experiences that facilitate the complex process known as learning.

It is often assumed that learning is a simple matter of presentation and absorption of new information. Learning is rarely seen as a process. Like many other human interrelationships it is lived with and dealt with daily, but it is seldom regarded as a matter to be studied or subjected to the scientific procedures that have carried us so far in other spheres of life.

Teacher-education curricula are based on the assumption that learning is a lawful, predictable, teachable function. The knowledge we have about learning has been acquired in the same painstaking, carefully controlled kind of experimentation that has made possible the advances of the other sciences. It is composed of facts and principles about an important human process, and it deserves the same understanding as any other body of scientific knowledge.[3] The principles of learning can no more be suspended than any other scientifically derived understanding. They continue to operate whether we are aware of them or not. If we ignore them, we do so at the risk of making teaching haphazard and ineffective.

The traditional view of learning equates knowledge and education with the acquisition of facts obtained only in schools. One of the unfortunate correlates of this view is the belief that education is the acquisition of facts and the more a person knows, the more educated he is. Rosenstock and others[4] have revealed that knowledge alone does not indicate learning, and knowledge about health does not necessarily determine health behavior. Therefore, health professionals should view education not as a process of hammering in bits and pieces of information, but as a "social process" in which

2. Morris Keeton, "The Climate of Learning in College," *College and University Bulletin*, 15: 1-2, 5-6, Nov. 15, 1962.

3. Arthur W. Combs and D. Snygg. *Individual Behavior: A Perceptual Approach to Psychology*, New York: Harper and Row, 1959, p. 59.

4. Irwin Rosenstock. "Why People Use Health Services: A Health Service Research Report," *Milbank Memorial Fund Quarterly*, 44:109-111, July, 1966; Linus J. Dowell, "The Relationship between Health Knowledge and Practice," *The Journal of Educational Research*, 62:201-2, January, 1969. Godfrey M. Hochbaum, "Measurement of Effectiveness of Health Education Activities," *International Journal of Health Education*, 14:2, April-June, 1971; Lynford L. Keyes, "Health Education in Perspective: An Overview," Health Education Monographs, 31:13-17, 1972.

learning occurs *primarily* as a result of human interaction based on self-knowledge and self-understanding.

Education viewed in this way is not restricted merely to classrooms or formal educational settings. Instead, learning may occur in any setting and throughout a person's life as the result of continued interactions with others and life events. Much health education occurs outside the classroom.

This theory of learning does not denigrate the importance of school health education classes. Instead, it forces health teachers to evaluate the impact they may have on the health behavior of students in relationship to the other health education the students receive. In essence, the consequences of the human interaction between the student and the teacher increase in importance. The nature of the relationship should receive as much attention as the learning tasks.

Readers can easily identify with this approach to the education process. Each of us can remember classes where subject matter, assignments, and tests were similar. In one class we strove to do our best and loved the course; yet, in the other class, we dreaded every moment. Why? Because of the teacher or medium through which we learned. As it was succinctly put by McLuhan, "the medium is the message." This example lends credence to the theory that learning is a social process too. "Simplistically put, we can say that the social interactions (medium) provide impact, not solely the subject matter (content)."[5] Therefore, educators in the area of health behavior need to examine both the subject matter and the social interaction in the educational process. Not only what message we send but also how we send it to the patient is important.


## Meaning and Learning

Today the big word in education is *relevance*. It is a favorite word among students. However, this word does not imply a new concept to educators. Dewey, Rogers, Combs, Snygg, and many others have expressed the same concept. Their words may have been different, but essentially they all spoke of relevance.

> *Significant learning is that learning which has*
> *meaning and importance to the life of the learner. To*
> *have meaning and importance, what is learned must*
> *affect that person's life or his potential to live life.*
> *Such learning usually occurs through human*

5. Combs and Snygg, *op. cit.*

*interaction, because we derive meaning from our relationships with other humans. . . . It's not that one person tells another the meaning of something, but instead that meaning is derived from the reaction of the persons involved.*[6]

The meaning and importance of any information supplied to students will affect their behavior only to the degree to which it has personal meaning or relevance to them. Therefore, diagnosing the educational need and the meaning of the health information message to the student is an important process in developing a health education program. One of the shortcomings of teachers has been that we have not given sufficient attention to the individual's perceptions. We have been concerned with showing a film or pamphlet that has meaning and importance in our own eyes, not in the student's. But to be effective, education for health must operate on these very personal levels of learning

## Self-Knowledge and Self-Understanding

A basic principle of education as a social process of human interaction is the importance of self-knowledge and self-understanding. "Self-knowledge refers to a knowledge of one's needs, behavioral tendencies, and values."[7] Self-understanding of personal motives enables the individual to become self-directed through informed choice rather than acting according to rote or habit or in response to directions from an authority figure.

Non-process-oriented educators are known for their absolute attention to the subject matter and complete disregard for the learners, except for their ability to parrot facts. Educational psychologists tell us that perhaps the single most important factor in leading an effective life is "an adequate self-concept based on accurate knowledge and understanding."[8] With knowledge of "self," individuals are more likely to behave in a manner that is beneficial to themselves.

An understanding of how patient / learners see themselves is imperative to the learning process. Remedial teachers know that most academic deficiencies are traceable to negative concepts of self, which in turn are derived from negative experience. Children and many adults carry self-perceptions of themselves as "dumb," "a slow

6. Gene Stanford and Albert E. Roark, *Human Interaction in Education,* Boston: Allyn and Bacon, 1974, p. 4.
7. Ibid., p. 3.
8. Ibid., p. 5.

learner" or "a person who can't do things as well as everyone else." Individuals with negative self-concepts are poor learners. The methods and materials may be of the latest technology, but if the learner is negative to his "self," little progress will be made.

Since self-concept is learned, negative self-concepts can be unlearned and replaced by positive self-regard. This means that attention to the self-concepts and self-understanding of the students must be built into any health education program, and it must be a part of the teacher's philosophy of education.

## Some Principles of Learning

The modern instructor is confronted with the difficult task of selecting and applying those concepts of learning that seem most personally satisfying, philosophically consistent, and educationally sound. Most teachers may eventually develop a psychology of learning that is actually a composite of many theories. Such an approach characteristically has been described as eclectic.

Despite the confusion, which is still very much apparent concerning the learning process, certain basic relationships have emerged and have been generally adopted in recent years. The following principles are among the more prominently accepted in keeping with modern educational psychology. Learning is most effective when:

The learning objectives and philosophy of the program are planned and clearly understood by both the instructor and the students.

Reciprocal respect and a friendly emotional atmosphere exists between the instructor and the students.

Students have meaningful, satisfying, and realistic goals that guide their learning activities.

Motivation is provided through a regard for the needs, interests, problems, and concerns of the student.

An attractive, aesthetic, safe, and healthful environment is provided.

Students are carefully studied by the instructor and provision is made for individual differences.

The learning activities and experiences are supplemented and enriched by the use of related materials.

A tolerance for failure is developed through the provision of a backlog of successes.

Students engage in active, real-life experiences that are related to one another and to the problems of home, school, and community.

There is continuous and periodic student and program evaluation.

The need for improvement in the quality of learning rather than in the quantity has been pointed out by many authorities.

A teaching method helps to provide a vehicle for meeting the obligation of quality health education. Care should be taken that the teaching does not become the objective; rather, it should be the process towards achievement of the learning objective.

## INSTRUCTIONAL PROCEDURES

A multitude of teaching techniques and procedures are commonly used in education to motivate students and promote the most effective learning. The majority of these have a direct and potentially significant applicability to health education. This section of the handbook is designed to provide certain basic information on methodology that should prove helpful to the health instructor. It contains descriptions of nearly 200 learning opportunities, many with a "value" or "need" clarification orientation. The list is alphabetized for easy reference.

### Basic Instructional Criteria

Before any single teaching technique can be utilized effectively, certain basic criteria should be considered. The selection and use of a particular method or instructional procedure should adhere to sound educational principles, such as the following:

1.  Any instructional procedure should be regarded as an educational tool to facilitate definite learning and not solely to entertain.

2.  The technique should have appeal and interest to the student and be suitable to the maturity of the group.

3.  The method of presentation should be guided by the objectives of the health instructional program, the total college health program, the overall curriculum, and education in general.

4.  There should be adequate preparation on the part of the instructor and adequate time, proper equipment, and suitable facilities available.

5. The procedure should be flexible enough in its application to allow provision for individual needs and differences.

6. The technique should utilize or incorporate learning opportunities that assure significance in the thinking and behavior of the student.

7. The procedure should provide for growth through progression of activities and concepts.

## Learning Activities Used in Health Teaching

**ANECDOTAL RECORD:** A descriptive account of events, episodes, or circumstances in the daily life of the student. Basically, it is a device that makes it possible to preserve significant incidents and information concerning student behavior for subsequent review. The major purpose is to provide a clear perspective and reference to certain kinds of student behavior as observed through systematic observation and evaluation.

**ANECDOTE:** A brief narrative of an incident or event of special interest. It is often personal or biographical.

**ARTWORK:** A term used to describe, in general, the use of artistic talent in the creation of objects or materials. Creativity should be stressed in student work.

**BRAINSTORMING:** A technique valuable for the stimulation and generation of ideas and the facilitation of their expression. Literally, it is the use of the brain to "storm" a problem by the identification of all possible ideas relating to its solution. The purpose of the procedure is to promote a quantity of ideas bearing upon a particular subject. It involves cooperative thinking by groups toward the solution to a specific problem.

**BULLETIN BOARD:** A sheet of wood, masonite, celotex, cork, or similar material, usually set within a frame. Sometimes it is called a tackboard or pinning board. It may be used for displaying pictures, charts, posters, clippings, examples of student work, photographs, or other learning materials. It offers infinite possibilities for presenting visual materials and may be used in the classroom, corridor, library, office, cafeteria, study hall, auditorium, and other locations.

**BUZZ SESSION:** A group activity designed to facilitate the dividing of a large class into smaller groups for discussion purposes. Designated groups ordinarily are composed of from five to eight members, depending upon the size of the class. It can be effectively used to deal with difficult questions, problems, or controversial issues. It involves discussion for a limited period of time and is sometimes called a subdiscussion or cluster group.

**CAPTIONLESS PICTURE:** A picture without printed or written description. Selected pictures are viewed by the class, and students are then asked to develop an appropriate caption or title for the illustration.

**CARTOON:** A form of comic art that can be used to depict important events, personalities, or circumstances. It presents a stimulated, but usually easily recognized and popular, graphic illustration of selected behavior or activity.

**CASE STUDY:** Entails the use of detailed studies of individual situations as a basis for instruction and the development of principles of action. It is based upon a thorough investigation of a case in order to shed light upon the background, conditions, circumstances, and other influences and relationships. True experiences of the instructor, student, or another person or a fictitious situation pertaining to a given subject may be utilized.

**CASSETTE:** A type of tape recording used to preserve sound. It is the smallest of those available and has the advantage of rewinding. It frequently is commercially produced to accompany filmstrips.

**CHALKBOARD:** A smooth surface, usually fastened to the wall or enclosed in a type of frame, on which one prints, writes, or draws with chalk. Unlike the slate blackboard of former years, the modern chalkboard may be found in green, grey, blue, or another pastel color. It is located in most classrooms as well as other instructional settings. The chalkboard is one of the oldest and most important forms of instructional aids.

**CHART:** A material upon which is placed visual symbols that may be used to summarize, contrast, compare, or explain subject matter. Charts reflect a wide range of interests and are commonly referred to by type, such as narrative, skill development, creative expression, reference, experience, teacher-composed, informational, or guidance. They represent one of the oldest forms of teaching, having been used even before languages developed.

**CHECK LIST:** A device used to determine the existence of certain conditions or circumstances. It is ordinarily developed to provide specific information on student behavior, some aspect of program, or certain qualities of an existing situation. It is completed by merely checking a statement or characteristic that has been determined to be important for evaluation. Published check lists are available in many areas of instructional concern, and lists may be constructed by the teacher or student.

**CLARIFYING RESPONSE:** A manner of responding to a student that results in a consideration of what has been chosen, what is prized, and / or what is being done. The approach encourages thinking about alternatives and the clarification of values.

**COLLECTION:** Materials, gathered individually or by a group, that relate to a particular topic or subject. The materials may consist of pictures, maps, clippings, letters, charts, books, stamps, leaves, and other similar specimens or objects. Collected materials are usually arranged in some sequence or order.

**COLLOQUIUM:** Involves the use of two panel groups — one consisting of authoritative resource persons and the other of selected class members. It permits direct class participation on an equal status with the invited "experts." A moderator is ordinarily utilized to guide the discussion, direct pertinent questions, and encourage panel and audience participation as desired.

**COMIC:** A form of pictorial art pertaining to comedy as distinct from tragedy. It is ordinarily developed to be amusing and to provoke laughter.

**COMMITTEE WORK:** Involves the active participation of individual class members in small group activity. A committee ordinarily consists of from four to twelve or more members and frequently explores phases of a particular problem or topic through the problem-solving approach. It is usually an on-going type of experience that may culminate in a project over a designated period of time.

**CONTRACT LEARNING:** A contract is an agreement between two or more parties for the doing or not doing of some definite thing. In contract learning the student contracts for a grade on the basis of the fulfillment of some predetermined assignments.

**CONTRIVED INCIDENT:** A situation developed to exaggerate circumstances in order to shock students into an awareness of what they are for or against. Its purpose is to simulate as closely and dramatically as possible something that will provide a real feeling, experience or understanding.

**CREATIVE WRITING:** A type of composition involving some degree of self-initiative, spontaneity, and exercise of the imagination by the writer. It may take various forms, such as short stories, verse, and drama.

**CRITICAL LISTENING:** Involves the use of skillful judgment as to the truth or merit of a particular assertion or reactions to the spoken word or other audio presentations. Health advertisements lend themselves well to such critical analysis.

**CURRENT EVENT:** Concerned with immediate or recent happenings that may be expressed through various means of communication. It includes circumstances as reported through newspapers, periodicals, popular magazines, radio, television, interviews, or other informative sources. Current events serve as a medium for relating local, state, national, or global occurrences to an understanding of everyday life.

**DEBATE:** Consists of a clear-cut pro and con discussion of a question or issue. It is conducted according to a definitive set of rules that is closely followed by the participants. It groups several speakers on each side that have a definite responsibility to perform in support of, or in opposition to, a given proposition. It actually is a specialized form of persuasion dealing with some specific resolution.

**DEMONSTRATION:** A process of graphic explanation of a selected idea, fact, relationship, or phenomenon. It involves the use and manipulation of materials and provides a visual experience that is usually increased in value by verbal explanation. The demonstration generally is utilized with a group of observer-participants by someone who is an expert on the given subject. It centers attention upon processes, relationships, or reactions that result from a skilled manipulation of objects, machines, or appliances.

**DEVIL'S ADVOCATE:** A productive strategy designed to stimulate the examination of alternatives to the solution of a problem. It often involves a strong stand against or for a particular issue that is not in keeping with popular opinion.

**DIAGRAM:** A figure or set of lines or marks to give the outline or general features of an object. It also may be used to show the course or results of a process.

**DIARY:** A book used for keeping a daily record. It usually is used to record personal experiences or observations.

**DISCUSSION:** Involves the verbal interaction of a number of individuals who perceive one another as participants in a common activity. It is a socializing procedure designed to utilize cooperative oral participation toward the resolution of a particular problem or question. A discussion may proceed with or without active leader direction, although some degree of moderation is usually necessary to effectively guide group thinking.

**DISPLAY:** To show, exhibit, or make something visible. A display may be used to carry out a theme, to simplify, or to summarize an idea.

**DRAMATIZATION:** An acted out presentation of an event, episode, situation, or story.

**EXHIBIT:** A display of materials that informs the observer about a subject of educational significance. It usually provides a realistic impression through the use of three-dimensional objects rather than flat materials. An exhibit may include posters, pictures, charts, graphs, specimens, and objects and may also incorporate recordings, films, slides and other audio or visual materials.

**EXPERIMENT:** A test, trial, or tentative procedure. It is an act or operation conducted to discover something unknown or to prove a principle.

**FIELD TRIP:** A visit to some location other than the normal classroom for educational purposes. Confirmatory field trips serve as a reinforcement for previously acquired learning, and exploratory excursions fulfill the basic function of discovery. Each approach is a structured attempt to provide an on-the-spot observation of some specific process, undertaking, or activity.

**FILM:** The film, or motion picture, is a sequence of photographs, pictures, or drawings that create an optical illusion of movement when projected on a screen in rapid succession. The motion picture encompasses visualization with or without color, music, narration, or sound relationships. It is a method of transmitting stimuli and experiences by recreating events, situations, or circumstances through action.

**FILMSTRIP:** A related sequence of transparent still pictures or images on a 35mm film which are projected in progression on a screen. It may be produced in black and white or in color and is sometimes accompanied by recordings of narration, music, and sound effects. The filmstrip typically consists of from twenty to fifty frames or pictures that may contain captions or titles.

**FLANNEL-FELT BOARD:** A piece of heavy cardboard, plywood, or other stiff material tightly covered with flannel or felt cloth to which objects treated with a sensitive backing may be attached. The materials to be displayed on the board may be backed with sandpaper, blotter material, felt, flocked paper, styrofoam, flannel, or a similar substance.

**FLIP CHART:** A series of pictures and / or statements arranged in sequence with a separate page for each new idea. It is bound so that each new page can be "flipped" over the last. It is helpful in showing a series of events or steps in logical progression.

**FORUM:** Consists of two or more presentations to a group on the same subject, with audience participation. It may be used to present opposing sides of a controversial issue and is followed by a question-and-answer period. It differs from debate in that no attempt is made to discredit a particular viewpoint. It considers all aspects of the question.

**GAME:** An educational play situation possessing some structure by virtue of a set of rules or procedures to be followed. Games may require varying degrees of skill, concentration, movement, and coordination, depending upon their organization and execution.

**GRAB BAG:** A bag containing objects or slips of paper with words or short phrases. Students reach into the bag and then describe the object or feelings about the words selected.

**GRAPH:** Involves various levels of visual expression ranging from a simple presentation of information to the most abstract statistical analysis. Graphic presentation serves the major functions of providing a concise summary, indicating a comparison, showing a relationship, or otherwise explaining a concept or idea.

**GUEST SPEAKER:** Sometimes referred to as an outside speaker or resource person. It is an individual who is invited to talk to a group on a given subject. The person usually is selected because of some special knowledge or talent that classifies her or him as an expert or an authority in the field.

**GUIDANCE:** A form of systematic assistance to help students assess their abilities, capabilities, and limitations in order to learn more effectively. The approach involves a dynamic interpersonal tionship designed to influence the ultimate behavior of the individual. It can be carried out individually or in groups.

**HANDOUT:** The distribution of materials to students. These usually consist of mimeographed papers, leaflets, pamphlets, or similar materials.

**HEALTH FAIR:** Consists of selected displays or demonstrations on different aspects of health and well-being. Students frequently plan, prepare, arrange, and manage the fair activity.

**INDEPENDENT STUDY:** Learning without undue influence from others. It generally is autonomous, or free, study without another's authority or jurisdiction. Some degree of guidance, however, is recommended.

**INTERVIEW:** A face-to-face procedure designed to elicit information outside the classroom which is related to current study. Interviews of appropriate individuals are frequently conducted by a single student or in groups of not more than three students and reported back to the class in summary form. Teachers also use the interview technique with students, parents, and others.

**INVENTORY:** A device or instrument used to ascertain the status of an aspect of student behavior, school or community activity, or instructional program. It frequently involves the gathering of information by means of self-appraisal procedures. Many standardized instruments are available, or the inventory may be teacher- or student-constructed.

**INVESTIGATION:** Means to follow up or research something. It involves inquiry, observation, and a close examination of facts.

**LABORATORY EXPERIMENTATION:** Involves an operation or series of tests undertaken to discover an underlying principle or to prove or disprove a specific point. It generally attempts to demonstrate how things are done, how they work, or some known truth. It involves experimental study for the purpose of illustration.

**LEAFLET:** A sheet of small pages that are folded but not stitched or taped together. Leaflets are available on most areas of health education.

**LECTURE:** Involves the formalized presentation of information by the teacher through oral exposition. It utilizes certain essential facts or basic information to impart knowledge, create interest, influence opinion, stimulate activity, or promote critical thinking. It frequently is supplemented by related teaching aids or instructional materials and proceeds with a minimum of class participation and interruption.

**LECTURE-DISCUSSION:** Incorporates the desirable qualities of both the lecture and the discussion into a formal technique. It consists of a verbal form of presentation with provision for clarification and further enlightenment through class participation and intergroup exchange.

**LIBRARY WORK:** Involves planned investigation into additional sources of information on a given topic or problem. Classroom, school, and community libraries provide a ready resource for research. Such reference sources might include encyclopedias, dictionaries, newspapers, books, pamphlets, atlases, magazines, almanacs, and other materials.

**LOOP FILM:** A short length of film spliced into a circle. The film is threaded into a projector and shown continuously without rewinding. Special loop film projectors are available. This process of repetition is especially valuable in emphasizing key points, illustrating basic skills, and demonstrating ideas that are difficult to learn.

**MAGNETIC BOARD:** A board constructed of metal or containing metal to which a magnet will adhere. It is especially useful in diagraming set procedures. Magnets may also be used through cardboard to depict motion.

**MANIKIN:** A model of the human body, usually in proportionate size. It is useful in learning about anatomy, physiology, artificial respiration, and other processes.

**MAP:** A representation, usually on a flat surface, of the face of the earth or some part of it. It shows relative size and position according to a scale, projection, or represented position. Various types of maps can be used in the classroom (e.g., contour, relief, dot, crosshatch, and pin maps). Maps can be used to illustrate physical, political, social, commercial, or economic dimensions.

**MOBILE:** A set or series of objects that are delicately balanced and suspended from a central point on string, fine wire, or thread in such a way as to sway with air movements. It is commonly constructed in a counter-balanced multiple form that rotates within itself and as a total assembly.

**MOCK-UP:** A scale model of a real object or a part of the object. It alters the elements of the original object, often simplifying or exaggerating details, to concentrate only on certain aspects in order to make them more understandable. Mock-ups are commonly used to understand complex processes, such as engines or functions of the human body.

**MODEL:** A recognizable three-dimensional imitation or replica of real objects, principles, or ideas. It usually is identical to the original in most respects except size and incorporates the essential features of the object or procedure.

**MONTAGE:** A picture made by arranging into one composition pictorial elements borrowed from several sources so that the elements are both distinct and blended into a whole. Superimposition is often used.

**MURAL:** A drawing or painting affixed to a wall. It usually depicts a scene or description of a particular event or circumstance.

**OBSERVATION:** Basically, the act of noticing and perceiving. Observations can be made in formal and informal settings by the teacher or students.

**OPAQUE PROJECTOR:** A device that utilizes reflected light to project nontransparent flat materials on a screen. It consists of a large metal box, bright illuminating lights, a blower to prevent the accumulation of excessive heat, a focusing lens, and mirrors that are arranged in such a manner as to magnify and reflect the materials being shown. It also may possess a built-in pointer and a rotating platform to facilitate the viewing of materials that have been arranged in a sequence.

**OPEN-END TECHNIQUE:** Consists of a partially stated question or statement to be completed by the student. It provides for an opportunity to reveal certain attitudes, beliefs, activities, or other "value indicators."

**OPPOSING PANELS:** A variation of the panel discussion technique. Panels are appointed to deal with the pros and cons of a particular issue. Different points of view are expressed through discussion.

**ORAL REPORT:** Refers to information that is verbally communicated by the student to the class. It is easily assigned and should be presented in relation to scheduled classroom work. Materials, such as charts, pictures, slides, photographs, and graphs, lend value and sophistication to the report and should be encouraged.

**OUTLINE:** A general sketch of a book, project, event, or subject. It is designed to indicate only the main features or key ideas.

**OUTSIDE READING:** Assigned reading in references other than those used in the classroom. Many resources might be assigned for such reading, such as paperback books, periodicals, newspapers, popular literature, and basic reference materials.

**OVERHEAD PROJECTOR:** A device that reproduces an image on a screen by way of light reflection from a mirror through any transparent material. Important advantages of the overhead projector are that it can be operated by the instructor from the front of the room and with the lights on.

**PANTOMIME:** A variation of role playing, sociodrama, and similar dramatic techniques. It differs in that gestures, facial expressions, and overt movements take the place of spoken words in the portrayal of character roles and situations. Sometimes an unobserved announcer is used to briefly describe the action as it occurs. It is a valuable way to demonstrate the "right and wrong" or "do and don't" of a situation that involves feeling and action.

**PAMPHLET:** A paperbound document, consisting of a limited number of pages, which is ordinarily devoted to a particular topic. The content is often restricted in scope and covers a given subject in detail. Many free and inexpensive pamphlets are available for educational use.

**PANEL DISCUSSION:** A conversational exchange of ideas by selected participants on a topic, problem, or issue. It is a relatively informal oral process that brings together individuals who possess differing points of view concerning a subject. It provides ample latitude for exploration and discussion. The group is commonly composed of from three to eight selected members who operate under the guidance and direction of a moderator. Opposing panels are sometimes utilized with question-and-answer exchanges.

PHOTOGRAPH: A picture produced by photography. Some newer camera equipment provides an almost instant reproduction.

PICTURE: Flat illustrative material, with little or no printed matter, that is used to provide a visual experience. It can be utilized in a variety of ways, such as displayed on bulletin boards, projected, or organized in booklet form. Pictures frequently are used to translate word symbols, enrich reading experiences, correct mistaken impressions, motivate activity, or stir the imagination.

PLAY: A carefully rehearsed dramatization that involves a predetermined script, costumed performers, and rather elaborate scenery. It can be extremely useful in vividly portraying important concepts, particularly those of a social nature. Play scripts are available in printed form from a number of sources or may be developed as a class project.

POSTER: A pictorial or symbolic visual representation designed to catch and hold the observer's attention long enough to implant a significant message or idea. It is intended to emphatically convey a single easily grasped idea. It stresses bold design, forceful color, clear organization, and careful word selection. It may vary from a simple printed card to highly artistic pictures and slogans. The use of the poster is many centuries old, having been utilized by early traders and merchants to advertise their wares.

PRE-TEST: A test given prior to instruction or evaluation. It serves to help establish basic levels of knowledge, attitudes, practices, interests, and other behavioral dimensions.

PROBLEM SOLVING: A complex integration of many kinds of responses that vary from one situation to another. It is not an isolated and unitary process but rather one that seeks new ways, modifications, and patterns of behavior for attaining a goal. It involves the presentation and analysis of a real or hypothetical problem to arouse curiosity, interest, and student activity that culminates in a scientifically determined conclusion or solution.

PROGRAMMED MATERIALS: A program is a plan to be followed. Programmed materials are designed to systemize learning by providing a sequential arrangement, usually progressing from simple to more complex. Such materials may be used with teaching machines.

PROJECT: Either an individual or class-planned undertaking designed to compile information, collect objects, construct materials, or create something. It is usually a task or problem, calling for constructive thought and action. As a group enterprise, a project might consist of such real-life experiences as creating a class newspaper. An individual learning opportunity, a project might involve painting a mural or writing a story.

**PROJECTION:** Involves the use of a stimulus to encourage spontaneous and uninhibited discussion or reaction to social, personal, or real-life situations. It is used to reveal attitudes, beliefs, ideas, and adjustments related to specific problems. Open-end or association techniques often are utilized as stimuli, such as completing a sentence or story, responding to a word or phrase, or describing a picture or symbol.

**PSYCHODRAMA:** The unrehearsed and spontaneous acting out by an individual of a personally perplexing problem. It has been successfully used as a diagnostic and therapeutic device for understanding and dealing with mental and emotional problems. It has educational value in helping to resolve personal conflicts and in demonstrating appropriate responses to problems.

**PUBLIC INTERVIEW:** An interview of an individual student conducted by the teacher in front of the class. It probably should be used sparingly.

**QUESTION AND ANSWER:** Is ordinarily utilized in a discussion-type setting. It may be carried out by the class under teacher or student direction or used in conjunction with resource persons. It is especially valuable in understanding new or technical information. It is frequently involved as a part of other learning procedures.

**QUESTIONNAIRE:** A well-known and frequently used type of survey form. It is commonly utilized to facilitate student opinion studies, self-appraisal procedures, or surveys of a particular curricular activity. Questionnaire results often are used in planning individualized programs to meet specific individual and group needs.

**QUIZ:** A short, sometimes informal test. It involves an examination of some dimension of student behavior and may be administered orally or in written form.

**QUOTATION:** That which is quoted or taken from another source. Usually consists of a passage from a book, speech, magazine, or other reference. Many compilations of quotations on various subjects are available.

**RAP SESSION:** An informal but intense discussion of feelings and opinions about a particular subject or issue. It is useful in highlighting fears, misconceptions and negative feelings about someone or something.

**RATING SCALE:** A device that is used for recording the judgments of observations. When properly developed and used, it helps to make subjective estimates of a situation, ability, or skill more objective. It can be effectively used in many different areas of evaluation and may be constructed for specific purposes.

**READING ASSIGNMENT:** Reading assignments enable the learner to journey beyond the confines of the classroom. They may merely involve perusal of a single textbook or go beyond into the vast world of supplementary printed materials. The use of multiple textbooks, typical reference volumes, current media, and student-teacher created materials have value as resources for basic or supportive reading.

**RECORDING:** A device used to record or duplicate sound. It may consist of a disk, cylinder, tape, or wire upon which sound has been recorded. The sound is then reproduced by playing the recording on a machine designed for that purpose. The phonograph record, tape recording, transcription, and recording disk are common examples. Recordings help to enrich learning and increase student listening skills.

**REPORT BOOK:** An account of an investigation into a topic, presented in book form. It is a detailed report of what has been learned by observation or research.

**RESOURCE PERSON:** Someone with expertise or experience in a particular field who is invited to speak or discuss a topic. Sometimes referred to as an outside, or guest, speaker.

**REVIEW:** Entails the reexamination or reevaluation of material previously presented or studied. It involves an overview of a unit of work or body of material in an attempt to identify the most important ideas and concepts. It represents a guided effort to facilitate clarity of understanding and the formulation of final generalizations. A variety of related techniques is commonly used in the review session.

**RHYME:** Represents a creative writing experience involving the manipulation of words to produce a form of rhythmic meaning. When used sparingly and with discretion, the approach provides personal satisfaction, serves to emphasize important points, and motivates the development of certain basic writing skills.

**ROLE PLAYING:** The spontaneous, unrehearsed, and on-the-spot acting out of a situation, incident, or specific problem. It is a form of improvisation in which the participants assume the identity of other persons and then react as they perceive their behavior in a particular set of circumstances. Spontaneity and invention characterize role playing with an emphasis upon individual performance and the role itself, rather than a coordinated group experience centered on the problem. Most effective role playing situations grow out of problems concerned with people, their beliefs, their feelings, and their actions.

**SCRAPBOOK:** A collection of pictures, articles, photographs, or other appropriate materials pertaining to a particular subject and placed together in a book. It enhances the ability to plan, collect, arrange, organize, and illustrate.

**SELF-APPRAISAL:** A technique requiring the individual to appraise personal strengths and weaknesses. It may utilize checklists or rating scales. Personal health practices, such as eating habits, growth and development characteristics, and immunization, are frequently assessed.

**SELF-TEST:** A series of questions, exercises, or other means of measuring personal skill, knowledge, attitudes, or other aspects of behavior. The self-testing instrument or device may be student or teacher constructed or in some instances standardized, but in each case it is administered by and to the individual personally. Sometimes the student competes against his previous record, as in certain activities, or against norms established individually, for the class, or even nationally.

**SEMINAR:** A small group of students engaged in a specific study. It is particularly useful with gifted students who are participating in advanced study or original research.

**SENSITIVITY TRAINING:** Sensitivity is simply a state or quality of being sensitive to others. Various degrees of training help to facilitate the process.

**SKIT:** A relatively brief dramatic presentation. It is frequently designed to provide a learning opportunity through a planned and rehearsed satirical, comic, or humorous story. It is often used as a tool in the exploration of problems in human relations.

**SLIDE:** Two- by two-inch photographic slides have largely replaced the lantern slide in many schools, although each has certain advantages for projection purposes. Slide projectors with automatic devices enable a greater flexibility for the teacher.

**SOCIODRAMA:** An unrehearsed and spontaneous dramatization dealing with some problem or issue of significance in a social relations situation. Sociodrama is characterized by attention to social problems that are acted out by the group.

**SOCIOGRAM:** A chart-type device that indicates certain relationships between individuals in a group at a particular time and under a given set of circumstances. It is designed to elicit responses that might be used to foster a greater understanding of individual problems and class attitudes, practices, and interactions.

**SOUND-ON-SLIDE:** A disk, developed by the 3M Company, to record sound and at the same time incorporate a visual slide. Each unit provides space for the insertion of a specific two-by-two slide and the recording of verbal description. A special sound-on-slide machine is required.

**STORYTELLING:** An intimate form of presentation, involving narration to a class, of material that possesses a plot. The story may be true or fictional, and it may be read, told, or presented through various forms of expression. Storytelling is an old and beautiful art that has been practiced for centuries. Its general aim is to present a message, interpret the literature, or inspire reading and expression.

**STRENGTH BOMBARDMENT:** A game-type situation that serves to help expose certain feelings of individuals in relation to the group. One student is "it" and sits in the center of a circle. Each member in turn describes what he or she likes about the one who is "it" and thus expresses only positive feelings.

**SURVEY:** Involves the investigation and study of specific problems or circumstances by means of a scientific process. It consists of measurement of personal or social attitudes, ideas, or practices from which a scientific analysis and evaluation can be made. It is frequently used to study individual or group practices, current program status, or the interrelationships of social process.

**SYMPOSIUM:** Consists of two or more relatively brief presentations to a group that deal with different specific phases of the same general subject or topic. The presentations are usually followed by some audience participation in the form of questions or discussion.

**TAPE RECORDING:** A tape upon which sound has been recorded by means of a special machine (tape recorder). The sound is then reproduced by playing the tape on a tape player. Reel-to-reel, cassette, and track tapes are available.

**TEACHING MACHINE:** A device that utilizes programmed materials for instructional purposes. It involves a fusion of learning and testing through a series of questions and answers presented in printed sequence on frames. The technique serves to organize subject matter into small steps and arranges them in a logical and cumulative progression from simple to more difficult.

**TEAM TEACHING:** A team is a number of persons associated in some joint action. In education such teaching consists of two or more instructors working together to facilitate learning.

**TELEVISION:** A device used to receive the reproduction of a scene or picture. This is accomplished by a means of converting light rays into electromagnetic waves and reconverting the waves into visible light rays. Educational television, through normal or closed-circuit procedures, is receiving increasing attention as an instructional method. Videotape recording makes it possible to preserve "master" shows for subsequent viewing and listening.

**TEST:** A test, commonly called an examination or quiz, is a device or procedure used to measure ability, achievement, attitude, interest, understanding, or other aspect of behavior. It may be objective or subjective in its measurement. There are numerous types of tests, such as those designed to indicate aptitude, appreciation, comprehension, character, cooperation, deduction, intelligence, knowledge, and personality.

**TEXTBOOK:** A book written on a particular topic with a definite focus on specific subject matter. Some textbooks have manuals and test questions for teacher use on the material included.

**THEME:** A paper developed by students on a particular topic or issue. It facilitates in-depth investigation, organization of information, and desirable conclusions or solutions to a problem.

**THOUGHT SHEET:** A paper or card submitted by a student indicating the thoughts that occupied attention during a given period of time. It should be written after due reflection and indicate something of a quality of living or thinking.

**TIME DIARY:** A chart of activities engaged in over a given period of time, broken down into half-hour or hour segments. It is similar to any other type of diary.

**TOUR:** The same as the field trip or excursion, although sometimes it is envisioned as of shorter duration. A walking tour close to the school, utilizing a camera, might be an example.

**TRACK TAPE:** Basically, it refers to the eight-track tape used to record songs and other audio material. Most commercial tapes consist of four basic programs with several items on each.

**TRANSPARENCY:** A transparent piece of plastic upon which visual or printed material is placed. It is then projected on a screen by reflected light via the overhead projector.

**TUTORIAL:** Instruction provided an individual student or students in very small groups. Special attention usually is given to personal interests, problems, and abilities.

**VALUE CONTINUUM:** A technique that provides for a full visual range of possibilities or alternatives on a particular issue. It involves the graphing of two polar positions with a range of thinking between each.

**VALUES CLARIFICATION TECHNIQUES:** Teaching techniques concerned with the process by which students can identify and clarify their existing values related to their health. Various classroom activities for individuals and small groups may be used. In some ways the teaching techniques are similar to teaching activities used in "Civics" or "Problems of Democracy" or "Problems of Living" classes in school social studies departments.

**VITAL STATISTICS:** The term refers to life, while *statistics* is the science of the collection and classification of data on the basis of relative occurrence or number as a foundation for induction. Vital statistics incorporate data concerning birth, death, disease incidence, and other aspects of health.

**WORKBOOK:** A book designed to guide the student by providing basic learning material in printed form. It ordinarily includes games, puzzles, self-test items, questions to be answered, and similar activities.

**WORKSHOP:** A group gathering in which individuals attack and study problems of such scope that they are of interest to most concerned. In a classroom setting, workshop activities are often specifically planned and organized by students and conducted under teacher guidance. The technique is also frequently used as an in-service improvement procedure for teachers, administrators, and other school personnel.

**VALUE SHEET:** Consists of a provocative statement and a series of questions duplicated on a sheet of paper and distributed to the class. The purpose is to raise an issue and to carry students through the value clarifying process.

**VIDEOTAPE:** Involves the use of a camera, monitor, and videotape equipment to preserve in picture and sound a particular event or situation. Instant replay is one of the greatest advantages of the technique.

# INVOLVING THE STUDENT

*Part One* ❧ *Chapter* **4**

## STUDENT PROJECT GUIDELINES

The purpose of student projects is to provide opportunity for individual learning experiences in a problem area that is currently relevant to the student. The requirements as to the type or number of projects should be determined by the instructor according to factors particular to each class situation. An activity is recommended. If some students elect to prepare a formal paper or complete a reading, they should get the instructor's approval. Alternate projects also should be cleared with the instructor before the student begins.

### Reporting Form for Activities

All reports should be typed or neatly handwritten.

Factual statements in outline form, anecdotal records, or chronological events are preferred to a formal presentation for reporting on activities.

Records or data collected should be included with the report.

The most important part of the report is the student's interpretation of his learning experience from his involvement with a chosen project, its value to him and to others.

### Grading of Student Projects

Some instructors prefer not to give grades for projects, since it is very difficult to compare projects or even to evaluate thoroughly any one individual project. It is advised that the evaluation be based on how well the student organized the project and achieved his objectives. A point or weight value for examinations, quizzes, course projects and class participation is advised.

Additional project ideas are included in the chapters in Part 2 of this handbook. Some items merely reflect possible discussion questions; others reflect participation.

## SUGGESTED STUDENT HEALTH PROJECTS

### Self-Improvement

Living without cigarettes.

Disciplining oneself to lose _____ pounds per week or per month to achieve the best weight for height and bone structure.

Exercising to maintain a high level of fitness.

Changing your eating habits and activities to gain _____ pounds per week or per month to achieve optimum weight for your height and bone structure.

Maintaining the desired weight if you have just lived through a reducing plan.

Relaxing and relieving tension from everyday routines and / or worrying.

Caring for skin or acne problems.

Overcoming loneliness or other personal problems.

### Visits to Various Community Health Organizations

Attend a lecture, panel, or other program on a health-related subject sponsored by a local community organization.

Attend Alcoholics Anonymous meetings. (There are local chapters in all major cities and suburban communities.)

Visit local convalescent homes or homes for the aged. Talk with the director or head nurse about health care problems of the aging, and the problem for the families (emotional, financial, etc.).

If there is a "Free Clinic" in your city, arrange a visit to learn what health problems are most frequently encountered.

## Service to Health Organizations or Individuals

Reserve Saturday afternoons to read to a blind child at a school for the blind, or to help him or her with homework, music lessons, or some other activity.

Volunteer as a recreation leader at one of the special schools for retarded or handicapped children.

If you play a musical instrument, entertain at a convalescent home or home for the aged on Saturday or Sunday afternoons.

Contact a tutoring agency and offer to help a child who needs remedial help.

Contact a local mental hospital and offer to be a regular visitor to play games and talk with young patients.

## Gathering Information

Conduct a survey or poll on views on a critical health issue.

Measure pollution at various spots in the community. Turn observations over to local health authorities, newspapers, and campus groups.

Interview local health officials in school or community health work. Make notes of services provided and the quality of care.

Wear a prosthetic aid or go blindfolded for a day. Record your feelings and problems (doors, steps, eating, dressing, how others react to you).

# THE METHOD OF READING
## REACTION[1]

As one reads, certain ideas or facts become significant while other ideas or paragraphs seem trivial. Occasionally a passage may even elicit a highly emotional response. In the reading method, the material is a stimulus to thought. It provokes one to react according to academic training, life experience, and maturity.

There are various ways of reacting to certain material. One can react to the validity of the evidence, the mode of presentation, or the content. The most common reading reaction is with reference to content. This commonly takes the specific incident that has special meaning. The following are examples of each type of reaction.

**FREE ASSOCIATION:** Includes anytning brought to mind by a given statement. It may evoke thoughts of past experiences, incidents, or observations. It may simply help to expound opinions or philosophical thoughts on the matter. The following is an example of free association.

*Stimulus Sentence* — "In addition we have mounted a gigantic campaign to persuade the public that there is a drug for every ill or misery — anxiety, depression, tension, and the physical symptoms associated with these, irritability, fatigue, lack of success in business, social life, in the family."

*Reading Reaction* — As I read this statement I had visual flashbacks to the commercials on television. During any evening the viewer will be told to take any number of different drugs, in addition to being persuaded to smoke several types of cigarettes. I have become so "fed up" with all these drug commercials that now whenever a commercial comes on, I immediately turn off the sound. The amusement which I get from watching the facial expressions of the actors seems to relieve any headache which I may have, gets rid of stomach gas, prepares me for sleep, relieves tension, cures my aching back, soothes my hot, tired feet, and turns me off cigarettes forever.

1.  Adapted from Herbert Jones, "Method of Reading Reaction."

**AGREE-DISAGREE:** One may agree or disagree with the author. In this approach, the stand should be supported with reasons and evidence, whenever possible. Mere assent or acquiescence is not enough. The following is an example of agreement supported by a personal reason:

*Stimulus Sentence* — "If the physician limits himself to clearing up symptoms, he doesn't necessarily cure the disease."

*Reading Reaction* — I agree with this immediately. It would seem that the real task would be to eliminate the cause rather than the overt behavior. I have thought of this often in connection with my YMCA camp work. I'm sure many of the boys that came to us from the detention home in Detroit had their delinquency checked while at camp, but I hardly feel that in two weeks we could remove the cause. I'm certain that this latent delinquency was stirred up once again when they were removed from the camp environment.

The following is an example of disagreement:

*Stimulus Sentence* — "When I ask parents how they account for delinquent behavior in their children, I usually receive the answer that it is the result of bad company and running around the streets."

*Reading Reaction* — This is true only to a certain extent. I believe that there are thousands of children who grow up under the same unfavorable circumstances and still show no signs of delinquency. Such conditions as bad company may provoke dissocial behavior, but it usually is not the underlying cause.

**SPECIAL INCIDENT:** Finally, reading material may remind one of some child, adolescent, or adult. The problems and adjustments of the students may apply to the statement at hand. The following example may clarify this type of reaction.

*Stimulus Sentence* — "Some children react aggressively to emotional deprivation."

*Reading Reaction* — This was, I feel, the key to the actions of Robert. He was a problem to most of the teachers in our school. If one looked into his background, he too had enormous problems. His mother had been married to, or lived with, numerous men so that neither Robert nor his sister knew their fathers. His sister, who was in the same class, was turning into a little tramp. This too was a sore spot with him. He would come striding into class looking like Picasso's "Rooster" with hostility in every step. He baited the teachers to get attention. For some reason I cannot fathom, Robert and I had few differences and quite often he helped me with classroom chores. I shall never forget the open-mouthed amazement of my homeroom when told that Robert had prepared all the equipment for a science project. He seemed quite happy about doing this, and sorry when the job was done. When Robert found a girl friend he tumbled head over heels in love. It meant so much to him who had been deprived for so long. I wish I could say that this was the end of my story . . . I wonder what the end will be.

This method is designed to help clarify thinking, gain a better understanding of others, and develop a sounder philosophy of health. Merely rephrasing what the author has said should be avoided. The student should be evaluated on the depth of response, insight, understanding, feeling, and sensitivity. After reading a paper, the teacher should know more about each student.

# READING REACTION FORM

CLASS: _____ NAME: _____

DATE: _____

TITLE: _____

_____

SUMMARY: _____

_____

_____

_____

_____

_____

_____

_____

_____

_____

_____

REACTION: _____

_____

_____

_____

_____

_____

_____

_____

_____

_____

_____

_____

_____

_____

# HOW TO WRITE YOUR CONGRESS OR
# SENATE REPRESENTATIVE

Representatives to Congress and the Senate get hundreds — even thousands — of letters daily from their constituents. Because letter writing is a key form of communication on the issues before the Congress, here are a few suggested dos and don'ts to assure that one's letter receives maximum attention:

If possible, send a typewritten letter on one side of a sheet of stationery.

Address the letter to Honorable John Doe, House of Representatives, Washington, D.C. 20515, Dear Mr. Doe; for Senators, Honorable John Doe, U.S. Senate, Washington, D.C. 20510, Dear Senator Doe.

In one or two sentences in the first paragraph, identify the subject of the letter, state the name of the bill together with its House or Senate bill number.

The second paragraph should contain reasons for writing about the bill—personal or professional experience provides the best supporting evidence. Be reasonable. Don't ask for the impossible. Don't threaten.

The third paragraph should ask the representative where he or she stands on the subject. Request a statement of position in the reply.

The fourth paragraph should express in one sentence your appreciation for the representative's attention to the letter and, if you like, for the representative's continuing service to your Congressional district or state.

Unless using professional or personal letterhead stationery, be certain your full name and address appears after the signature.

If you are pleased with the vote on an issue, write and tell the representative so. A large amount of the mail received is from displeased constituents.

The timing of a letter is important. If possible, write when the legislature is pending—in committee. However, sometimes the representative may reserve judgment—and the vote—until the sentiment of the constituency has crystallized.

Permission to adapt from the Council for Exceptional Children, Suite 900, 1411 South Jefferson Davis Highway, Arlington, Va. 22202. Additional pointers are available from the booklet *When You Write to Washington.* Individual copies may be obtained from the League of Women Voters Education Fund, 1730 M Street, N.W. Washington, D.C. 20036. 35ᶜ per copy.

# Part Two

Detailed information on behavioral
objectives, methodology, learning
materials, reading lists, and test
questions for class use are provided in
this section. Specific suggestions are
given for involving students and for
having them assume personal
responsibility for learning, both in a
cognitive way and in an affective way.

# Chapters ৵

# HEALTH CONCEPTS

*Part Two* ᥣ *Chapter* 5

---

### BEHAVIORAL OBJECTIVES

The Student

- defines health consistent with modern thought and practice

- identifies some of the factors that influence the well-being of the college student

- describes the major divisions of the health care system and the contributions of each

- lists current significant health problems that remain to be solved

- identifies the specific target groups in need of health education

# SUPPLEMENTARY TEACHING AIDS

## Films

*The Farm Workers in California,* color, 18 min. A documentary film of California farm workers presenting present-day conditions on some large modern California farms. The film presents harvesting of fruits and vegetables that appear in the supermarkets. The process is different from romantic concepts of life in the country. Association-Sterling Films, 600 Grand Avenue, Ridgefield, N.J. 07657

*The Heritage of Operating Room "D,"* color, 27½ min. A fascinating, touching film about the many advancements in surgery and anesthesiology that make it possible for physicians to repair three-year-old Lynda's heart. Narrated by a stage and screen actor, the wonders of modern-day surgery are unfolded. Modern Talking Pictures, 3 East 54th Street, New York, N.Y. 10022.

*Leo Beuerman,* color, 13 min. The impact of this film is such that the viewer must reexamine his health values and attitudes. Leo Beuerman's life shows determination and adaptation in overcoming problems common to all men regardless of their state of health. Centron Educational Films, Suite 625, 1255 Post St., San Francisco, Calif. 94109.

*Little Marty,* color, 5 min. The film highlights a day with Marty, age 8, born with no arms and a short leg. With artificial arms and a built-up shoe, he feeds himself, paints, types, swims, and plays ball, revealing great determination and courage. National Foundation, Public Ed. Division, 1275 Mamoroneck Avenue, White Plains, N.Y. 10602.

*Reston Today,* color, 15 min. Explosive population growth in the past twenty years has created ugly urban and suburban sprawl. Totally new and complete cities such as Reston, Virginia, a few miles from Washington, D.C., are an answer. Within ten years Reston has become a new home and place to work for 75,000 people. Association-Sterling Films, 600 Grand Avenue, Ridgefield, N.J. 07657.

*A Special Kind of Matter,* color, 28 min. From where does life originate? In this fascinating film, scientists tell of the substance prostaglandin: what it does, how it was discovered, and its relationship to most forms of life. Modern Talking Films, 3 East 54th Street, New York, N.Y. 10022.

*There Will Be a Slight Delay,* color, 28 min. America is being hard-hit by transportation problems. This interesting documentary explores the highways, airports, railroads, of our cities and exposes existing problems, as well as suggesting what may be done in the future. Modern Talking Pictures, 3 East 54th Street, New York, N.Y. 10022.

Transparency originals (See Part III of Handbook)

# ORGANIZATIONS THAT HAVE MATERIALS *

Association for the Advancement of Health Education, 1201 16th St., N. W., Washington, D.C. 20036.

American Health Foundation, Inc., 320 East 43rd St., New York, N. Y. 10017.

American Medical Association, Bureau of Health Education, 535 North Dearborn St., Chicago, Ill. 60610.

American Public Health Association, 1015 Eighteenth St., N. W., Washington, D.C. 20036.

American School Health Association, 107 Depeyster St., Box 416, Kent, Ohio 44240.

Brookings Institution, 1775 Massachusetts Ave., Washington, D. C. 20036.

Consumer Product Safety Commission, 5401 Westbard Ave., Room 100, Washington, D. C. 20207.

Hastings Center, 360 Broadway, Hastings on Hudson, N. Y. 10706.

National Center for Disease Control, Public Inquiries, 1600 Clifton Rd., N. E., Atlanta, Ga. 30333.

National Center for Health Education, Suite 2564, 44 Montgomery St., San Francisco, Calif. 94104.

National Health Council, 1740 Broadway, New York, N. Y. 10019.

World Health Organization, Office of Public Information, 505 Park Ave., New York, N. Y. 10022.

*The addresses of these organizations and their policies concerning the sending of materials are subject to change without notice.

---

## STUDENT INVOLVEMENT

### Investigations

Identify some of the factors that influence health, and discuss some of the personal and community measures that might be taken to bring about improved well-being.

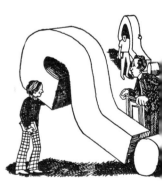

List the most significant health needs and problems of college age people. How can they best be alleviated?

Contrast health status and life expectancy statistics of today with years past and indicate some of the reasons for recent progress.

Individually select one important factor influencing health that might personally be improved, and develop a course of action leading to improvement.

What is meant by optimal well-being? How does this concept relate to personal patterns of living?

Investigate and obtain several different definitions of health, and attempt to identify the common elements found in each.

Summarize the number and types of student health and safety problems on campus as revealed through various college health and safety records.

Prepare a paper on consumer interest in "health" foods and "health" clubs.

## Action

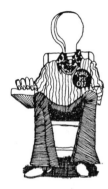

Prepare a debate on the topic of health care as a "right" for all citizens through a national health plan.

Conduct a community survey to determine citizens' opinion on government as the regulating agency against pollution by industry. Do people believe the government should strictly protect the environment and the public from injuries caused by industry?

Survey campus opinion on the statement, "Adequate health care is a right of every citizen."

Develop an "underground" type newspaper expounding the virtues of "good health" in all its dimensions. Include articles, drawings, cartoons, and other materials.

Listen to the record "In the Year 2525" by Zager and Evans. React to the record. What are the implications of the words? Is this real or imaginary?

## SOURCE MATERIALS

Barber, Bernard, "The Ethics of Experimentation with Human Subjects," *Scientific American*, 234: 25-31, February, 1976.

Black, Peter, "Focusing on Some of the Ethical Problems Associated with Death and Dying," *Geriatrics*, 31:138-41, January, 1976.

Blokker, J. William, "A 'Far Out' Philosophy of Health Education," *Health Education*, 6:29-30, November—December, 1975.

Brook, Robert H., and Kathleen Williams, "Quality of Care for the Disadvantaged," *Journal of Community Health*, 1:132-156, Winter, 1975.

Cohen, Toba J., "A New Approach to an old Curriculum: How Healthy Is Health Education?" *Today's Health*, 54:28-29, 50, January, 1976.

Edwards, Ralph, "Health and Medical Care at the Time of the American Revolution," *The Journal of School Health*, 46:19-23, January, 1976.

Hacker, Sylvia S., and Nancy S. Palchik, "Can Some Approaches to Health Education Become Hazardous to Health?" *Journal of the American College Health Association*, 23:121-123, December, 1977.

Hoyman, Howard S., "Models of Human Nature and Their Impact on Health Education," *Nursing Digest*, 3:37-40, September—October 1975.

Kahn, Carol, "The Golden Rule of Health," *Family Health*, 10:40-43, April, 1978.

Landsmann, Leanna, "Is Teaching Hazardous to Your Health?" *Today's Education*, 67:48-50, April-May, 1978.

Martin, Edward D., "The Federal Initiative in Rural Health," *Public Health Reports*, 90:291-97, July—August, 1975.

O'Connor, Robin, "American Hospitals, The First 200 Years," *Hospitals*, 50:62-72, January, 1976.

Petrello, Marjorie, "Your Patients Hear You, But Do They Understand?" *RN*, 39:37-39, February, 1976.

Phillips, Donald F., "American Hospital: A Look Ahead," *Hospital*, 50:70-85, January, 1976.

Remington, Richard D., "Blood Pressure, The Population Burden," *Geriatrics*, 31:48-54, January, 1976.

Sehnert, Keith, "But Has Medicine Forgotten the Patient?" *Family Health*, 7:60-61, November, 1975.

Simonds, Scott K., "Health Education Today: Issues and Challenges," *The Journal of School Health*, 47:584-593, December, 1977.

Slater, Philip, "Cultures in Collision," *Psychology Today*, 4:31-32, 66, 68, July, 1970.

Tritsch, Len, "School Health Education Today," *Health Education*, 7:5-6, January-February, 1975.

Weiss, Brian, "The New Archeology," *Psychology Today*, 8:50-58, May, 1975.

## TEST QUESTIONS

### Multiple Choice Items

1. The word *health* as currently envisioned denotes: (a) Absence of illness or disorder, (b) Maximal functioning of the body, (c) *A state of well-being resulting in effective*

*living,* (d) No physical or emotional defects, (e) A strong body.

2. The leading cause of death among the college-age population is: (a) Heart disease, (b) Suicide, (c) *Accidents,* (d) Cancer, (e) Tuberculosis.

3. The leading cause of death among the total population today is: (a) Arthritis, (b) *Heart and circulatory disease,* (c) Tuberculosis, (d) Cancer, (e) Nephritis.

4. Of the five leading causes of death among college-age students: (a) *Three have psychogenic components,* (b) Three could be retarded by periodic medical examinations, (c) There is little difference among the population as a whole, (d) One can be prevented by immunization, (e) All are communicable.

5. A sound, comprehensive college health program includes: (a) Innoculations, first aid, infirmary services, (b) *Health services, healthful environment, and health science instruction,* (c) Screening tests, sanitation, infirmary services, (d) Screening tests, instruction and sanitary facilities, (e) Vision screening, urinalyses, and first aid.

6. Today the concept of *healthy* must include the ability to: (a) Change the environment, (b) Change with the environment, (c) Resist unhealthy changes in the environment, (d) a and c, (e) *a, b, and c.*

7. In the current affluent society of the U.S., the heath problems for the majority of the people are caused by: (a) Poor medical services, (b) Poor-quality medical personnel, (c) *Personal health habits,* (d) Poor genetics.

8. Although hereditary traits are a contributing factor, an individual's health status is closely related to: (a) Religion, (b) Occupation, (c) *Overall life style.*

9. Current world health problems are most directly affected by: (a) Economic growth and industrialization, (b) *Population growth,* (c) Political structure, (d) Religion.

10. The "green revolution" of the sixties provided: (a) Unbelievable yields in grain crops around the world, (b)

*Disappointment in that gains in agriculture did not occur as expected,* (c) Additional income to millions of small farmers all over the world.

11. The average life expectancy in the United States for a child born in the late seventies is: (a) *70 years of age,* (b) 80 years of age, (c) 90 years of age.

12. Recent surveys of the public's knowledge about disease symptoms indicate that: (a) The public is fairly well informed about signs and symptoms of serious disease, (b) The older population is better informed about signs and symptoms of disease than the younger population, (c) *The public is generally poorly informed about signs and symptoms of serious disease.*

13. According to the definitions presented in Chapter 1, health may be perceived as: (a) *A condition that is dynamic and interrelated within each individual and his environment,* (b) The absence of disease, (c) The absence of any debilitating disease, either physical or mental, (d) A condition achieved by only a few individuals who obtain true optimality of potential within the physical, mental, emotional and spiritual domains.

14. There is a range and various levels of health. Theoretically, it ranges from zero health or death at one end of a continuum to the other end, which is best described as: (a) Wellness, (b) Soundness, (c) *Optimal health,* (d) Wholeness, (e) Health.

15. Health education currently is perceived by authorities in the field to be: (a) An integral part of physical education, (b) A subdivision of public health, (c) A specialty of medicine, (d) *A separate discipline,* (e) A part of anatomy and physiology.

**Essay Items**

1. The World Health Organization has defined health as a "state of complete physical, mental, and social well-being and not merely the absence of disease or infirmity." In addition, the organization has delineated four levels of public health for obtaining this health standard for the world. These four levels of public health are:

*LEVEL 1*   MORTALITY — encompasses the efforts to conserve life, as in the successful fighting of deadly plagues and famines.

*LEVEL 2*   SERIOUS MORBIDITY — the level at which efforts are made to prevent, control, and treat diseases and conditions that disable, cripple, or produce chronic illnesses.

*LEVEL 3*   MINOR MORBIDITY — the level at which efforts are made to control or alleviate minor illnesses and disturbances, such as the alleviation or control of smog, the common cold, tension, digestive disturbances, and adverse social conditions.

*LEVEL 4*   POSITIVE HEALTH — the level at which there is a complete control of health hazards.

Using the above information, and your knowledge of various concepts of health, *discuss the following questions.*

a. How does your definition and concept of health compare with the World Health Organization's definition? Would you omit certain phrases, add others, or emphasize certain parts?

b. Why and where are there various levels of health or health objectives?

c. What level (or levels) of health is of most concern to the average American? Compare this to the level of health of most concern to three other major areas of the world?

d. What means might quickly and efficiently bring countries such as those in Africa, Asia, or Latin America to higher levels of health? What problems might be encountered in improving the levels of health in specific countries?

e. How might our concept of healthful living change by the year 2050? What factors might influence this change?

2. Concepts related to health have changed over the years. Indicate and briefly discuss some characteristics of health in terms of modern day thought.

3. Many interrelated factors contribute to the total functioning of the individual. What are some of the prominent factors that influence health today?

4. Health problems may be indentified by various means. What are some of the major health problems of college students as demonstrated by morbidity and mortality statistics and by research studies of this population?

5. What are the moral and ethical implications of new medical advances such as life-support equipment, prenatal diagnosis of diseases, and long-term use of mood-altering drugs in therapy?

# HEALTH INFORMATION, PRODUCTS AND SERVICES

*Part Two* & *Chapter* **6**

## BEHAVIORAL OBJECTIVES

The Student

- analyzes the difference between a quack and a competent medical practitioner

- can identify questionable and fraudulent health practice

- indicates the more common areas of quackery and fraudulent health practice today

- states scientific criteria for the evaluation of health information and the selection of health products and services

- reports reliable and unreliable sources of health information as they relate to the selection of products and services

- distinguishes between various medical specialties and different health advisors

- categorizes different forms of medical care and provisions of each

- discusses some of the protective measures afforded the consumer and the agencies that provide such protection

## SUPPLEMENTARY TEACHING AIDS

*Consumer Education Bibliograph*, 1971, $1.60, Office of Consumer Affairs, Executive Office of the President, U.S. Government Printing Office, Washington, D.C. 20402. A comprehensive directory of consumer advising offices, governmental and private sources of consumer education materials, bibliography of current journal articles, books, pamphlets, films, filmstrips, posters, teaching games.

### Films

*The Health Fraud Racket*, color, 28 min., 1967. This film, which is still pertinent to the seventies, exposes the sly charlatan and his cunning traps of quackery in many areas of the health consumer's life. Distinguishes between fraudulent and legitimate products and explains how to combat being duped. U.S. Food and Drug Administration, Public Health Service, Audio Visual Facility, Atlanta, Ga. 30333. Free loan.

*Medicine Man*, color, 27 min. Prepared by A.M.A., the film exposes some of the prevailing errors of food fadism, using dramatic techniques to show modern "medicine man" at work selling his wares. Sterling Movies, Booking Dept., 43 West 61st St., New York, N.Y. 10023.

*To Seek . . . To Teach . . . To Heal*, color, 29 min. A multi-award winning documentary on the real efforts of medical personnel fighting to save the life of a three-year-old boy afflicted with a puzzling blood disease. Association-Sterling Films, 600 Grand Avenue, Ridgefield, N.J. 07657.

Transparency originals (See Part 3 of Handbook)

### Filmstrips and Slide Sets

*Dr. Quack's Lab*, 1970, color, 13 min., 40 frames. $4.50. A basic set revealing fraudulent medical devices that have been removed from the racket. U.S. Food and Drug Administration. Photo Lab, Inc., 3825 Georgia Avenue, N.W., Washington, D.C. 20011.

Kit — *Defenses Against Quackery*, pamphlets and reprints. American Medical Association, 535 North Dearborn St., Chicago, Ill. 60610.

*They Are Not Alone*, color, 15 min. Filmstrip with 33⅓ rpm record narration. This filmstrip offers an introduction to the subject of Public Health Nursing. It is designed to acquaint the viewer with the training and duties of the visiting nurse. Visiting Nurse Service of New York, 107 East 70th Street, New York, N.Y. 10021.

# ORGANIZATIONS THAT HAVE MATERIALS *

Aetna Life Insurance Company, Public Relations and Advertising Dept., 151 Farmington Ave., Hartford, Conn. 06115.

American Medical Association, Bureau of Health Education 535 N. Dearborn, Chicago, Ill. 60610.

Consumer Federation of America, 1012 14th St., N.W., Washington, D.C. 20005.

Consumer Product Information Center, Pueblo, Colorado 81009.

Consumers Union of the U.S., 256 Washington St., Mount Vernon, N.Y.

Educators Mutual Life Insurance Company, Lancaster, Pa. 17602.

Equitable Life Assurance Society of the U.S., Bureau of Public Health, 1285 Ave. of the Americas, New York, N. Y. 10019.

Food and Drug Administration, Department of Health, Education and Welfare, 5600 Fishers Lane, Rockville, Md. 20852.

Good Housekeeping Institute, 57th St. and Eighth Ave., New York, N. Y. 10019.

Metropolitan Life Insurance Company, 1 Madison Ave., New York, N. Y. 10010.

National Association of Blue Shield Plans, 840 North Lake Shore Drive, Chicago, Ill. 60611.

National Better Business Bureau, Inc., 405 Lexington Ave., New York, N. Y. 1001

National Consumers League, 1785 Massachusetts Ave., N.W., Washington, D.C. 20036.

Proctor and Gamble, Public Relations Division, Gwynne Building, Cincinnati, Ohio 45201.

Prudential Insurance Company of America, Public Relations and Advertising, Prudential Plaza, Newark, N. J. 07101.

Travelers Insurance Company, One Tower Sq., Hartford, Conn. 06115.

Underwriter's Laboratories, Inc., 207 East Ohio St., Chicago, Ill. 60611.

U.S. Consumer Product Safety Commission, Bureau of Education and Information, Washington, D. C. 20207.

U.S. Department of Agriculture, Consumer and Food Economics Institute, Washington, D. C. 20250.

*The addresses of these organizations and their policies concerning the sending of materials are subject to change without notice.*

# STUDENT INVOLVEMENT

## Investigations

Define what is meant by health consumer and discuss why it is of individual and public concern.

Are there loopholes in the present laws that provide legal protection against quackery and fraudulent medical practice? If so, what additional legislation might be recommended to alleviate these conditions? Follow up on one of your recommendations.

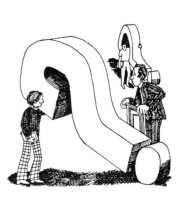

Discuss the statement, "Everyone is a Health Consumer."

Plan a sample family budget that provides for essential medical care, and discuss the value of prepayment health insurance. Compare it to your present personal or family health insurance plan.

Is the American consumer more or less "health educated" today than twenty-five years ago? How has the dissemination of health information changed within the past half century? What are the primary sources of health information for the average household?

Study the lives and operation of some of the famous quacks. Identify the common characteristics evidenced. Present a fifteen-minute "pitch" in class which demonstrates the techniques used by quacks. How many can the class then identify?

What is implied by the statement, "He who hath himself for a doctor has a fool for a patient"? What is meant by the term *activated patient*?

Collect clippings of testimonials on advertised products and indicate some of the ways that people might be influenced to purchase and use these health products.

What professional preparation and licensing is required for

osteopaths, dentists, podiatrists, nurses, pharmacists, physical and occupational therapists, clinical psychologists, therapists, and social workers?

Is the present-day chiropractor qualified to be a "family doctor"? Present current arguments for and against.

## Action

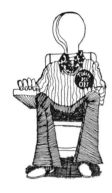

Make a tape recording of a series of radio or television commercials. Analyze the statements in class and develop some commonsense rules for critical evaluation.

Survey areas of a nearby county or city to determine availability of comprehensive health care facilities. Plot on maps. Are these facilities adequate for the needs of those residing in the areas?

Survey your campus for health superstitions and questionable health practices among college students. Example: Agree-Disagree item. The best first aid for a minor burn is to apply butter. What percentage of students polled agree, disagree with this statement and what was the source of their information?

Evaluate drug advertisements in medical journals. How are physicians influenced? On what basis should a physician prescribe drugs? How does the average family doctor learn about the use and availability of new drugs?

Survey health—hospital insurance plans and evaluate what plans are suited for a single person, young marrieds, middle-aged couples and the elderly. Present information to class.

Visit a "Free Clinic" and a Health Department Clinic. Compare type of treatment and effectiveness in meeting the needs of the community. Deliver your observation report to the Local Health Officer, newspaper, Medical Society, and other community groups who should be interested.

Visit your student health center. Evaluate effectiveness in meeting the needs of the students: Check the waiting time for appointments, referral services, amount of patient teaching or counseling, policy for handling venereal disease and pregnancy cases. Deliver your report to the campus newspaper and the Director of the Health Services.

Contact the local Health Board, Medical Society, Health Systems Agency or similar group. Request permission to attend meetings to observe proceedings. Report observations.

## BASIC SOURCE MATERIALS

Barrett, Stephen, "Health Frauds and Quackery," *FDA Consumer*, 19:12-16, November, 1977.

Brownlee, Ann Templeton, *Community Culture and Care*, St. Louis: Mosby, 1978.

Creighton, Lucy Black, "The Limits of Consumerism," *Social Policy*, 8:121-32, November-December, 1978.

"Fifteen Advertisers Drop or Change Ad Claims after Challenge," *Consumer Newsweek*, 5:2-3, January, 1976.

Gagnon, Jean, and Christopher Rodouskas, "The Influence of Wholesale Discounts and Other Factors on Prescription Ingredient Costs," *American Journal of Public Health*, 64:969-76, October, 1974.

Green, Lawrence W., "Constructive Consumerism," *Health Education*, 6:3-6, November-December, 1975.

Gumbhir, Ashok, and Christopher Rodouskas, "Consumer Price Differentials between Generic and Brand Name Prescriptions," *American Journal of Public Health*, 64:977-82, October, 1974.

Hall, Ross H., "The Food Fabricators," *Environment*, 18:25-34, January-February, 1976.

*Handbook of Non-Prescription Drugs*, Washington, D.C.: American Pharmaceutical Association, 1973.

Holbrook, Stewart H. *The Golden Age of Quackery*, New York: The Macmillan Company, 1969.

Horworth, Beckett, "Your Physician and You," *Consumer's Research Magazine*, 61:11-12, 18, April, 1978.

Jeffers, William, "Four Sharp Ways to Cut Your Life Insurance Costs," *Medical Economics*, 53:123-126, January, 1976.

Kushnick, Theodore, "When to Refer to the Geneticist," *Journal of the American Medical Association*, 235:623-25, February, 1976.

Manber, Malcolm, "The Medical Effects of Coffee," *Medical World News*, 17:63-73, January, 1976.

Map, Norman, "How Television Tries to Close the Health Information Gap," *Today's Health*, 54:31-33, 52, January, 1976.

Margolius, Sidney, "The Consumer's Real Needs," *The Journal of Consumer Affairs*, 9:129-38, Winter, 1975.

Rakstis, Ted J., "Sensitivity Training: Fad, Fraud, or New Frontier?" *Today's Health*, 48:20-25, 86-87, January, 1970.

Roalman, A.R., "Let the Buyer Be Aware," *Today's Health*, 48:66-67, 86-87, March, 1970.

Roghmann, Klaus J., et al., "Who Chooses Prepaid Medical Care," *Public Health Reports*, 90:516-27, November-December, 1975.

Rossman, Michael, "Warning: Consumer Education May Be Dangerous," *Social Policy*, 8:117-20, November-December, 1978.

Schmidt, Alexander M., "Dangerous Food and Drugs," *U.S. News and World Report*, 80:52-55, February 23, 1976.

Schonwalder, Christopher, and Annabel Hecht, "Aerosols, Ozone, and FDA," *FDA Consumer*, 9:5-7, September, 1975.

Smith, Ralph L., "Chiropractic: Issues and Answers," *Today's Health*, 48:64-69, January, 1970.

Solomon, Stephen, "The FDA: Help or Hindrance," *Family Health*, 10:34-37, 43, March, 1978.

Stellman, Jeanne M., "What Price Hearing," *Environment,* 17:29-31, September, 1975.

Steorts, Nancy, "Some Consumer Concerns Regarding Food Labeling and Packaging," *Food Technology*, 29:54-56, October, 1975.

"The Protected Consumer," *Consumer's Research*, 59:41, January, 1976.

"Your Health Insurance: Be Sure You Have What You Need," *Changing Times,* 31:45-47, June, 1977.

Warland, Rex, Robert Herrmann, and Jane Wellits, "Dissatisfied Consumers: Who Gets Upset and Who Takes Action," *The Journal of Consumer Affairs*, 9:148-163, Winter, 1975.

Weisinger, Mort, "Read Well before Taking," *Family Health*, 7:39, August, 1975.

White, Richard, "Making Blood Money Safe and Respectable," *FDA Consumer*, 9:11-19, January, 1976.

Wilson, F. Paul, and Alan Nourse, "The Controversy over National Health Insurance," *Social Education*, 40:88-92, February, 1976.

## TEST QUESTIONS

### Multiple Choice Items

1. A product distributed for sale by a health quack is termed a: (a) Testimonial, (b) *Nostrum,* (c) Proprietary, (d) Therapeutic, (e) Prescription.

2. Particularly susceptible to the wares and promises of the modern day quack and health charlatan are: (a) Infants, (b) Pre-school children, (c) Teenagers, (d) College students, (e) *The aged.*

3. Faddists and quacks make their claims for the following reasons: (a) They believe they have a good product or service, (b) They are after personal gain, (c) They are uninformed, (d) *Any or all of the above,* (e) None of the above.

4. Probably the best criterion for checking the accuracy of written medical and health information is: (a) *Its source and who said it,* (b) Where it was published, (c) How well it is documented, (d) How recently it was published, (e) The motive for publication.

5. The percentage costs of total income spent for health

care through the year is: (a) *Steadily rising,* (b) Staying about the same, (c) Slowly decreasing, (d) Greater for the rich than the poor, (e) Greater for the poor than the rich.

6. In 1965, Congress passed the "Medicare" bill to help meet the costs of medical care for people 65 years of age and over. The funds for the program come in large part from: (a) *Social Security taxes,* (b) Health Insurance Foundations, (c) Personal income taxes, (d) Blue Cross, (e) Treasury Department.

7. Which of the following health advisors is not licensed to treat diseases in the full sense of the term? (a) General practitioner, (b) Osteopath, (c) *Chiropractor,* (d) Internist, (e) Pediatrician.

8. What physician specializes in kidney conditions as well as problems relating to the male genital organs? (a) Otolaryngologist, (b) Neurologist, (c) *Urologist,* (d) Radiologist, (e) Gerontologist.

9. What physician has a medical degree, performs surgery, and treats diseases of the eye? (a) *Ophthalmologist,* (b) Optometrist, (c) Optician, (d) Chiropractor, (e) Otologist.

10. What physician specializes in treating diseases of the stomach and intestines? (a) Otolaryngologist, (b) Neurologist, (c) Internist, (d) Gynecologist, (e) *Gastroenterologist.*

11. The Food and Drug Administration has the responsibility of protecting the health and well-being of consumers of: (a) Foods and Drugs, (b) *Food, drugs, and cosmetics,* (c) Foods and cosmetics, (d) Drugs and cosmetics, (e) Foods.

12. The federal law controlling unfair competitive methods and false advertising is administered by the: (a) Federal Security Agency, (b) United States Public Health Service, (c) Food and Drug Administration, (d) *Federal Trade Commission,* (e) United States Department of Commerce.

13. What physician specializes in treating disease of the ears, throat, sinuses, and nose: (a) Pediatrician, (b)

Internist, (c) *Otolaryngologist*, (d) Orthopedist, (e) Radiologist.

14. What physician specializes in disease of the bones and joints? (a) Pediatrician, (b) Internist, (c) Otolaryngologist, (d) *Orthopedist*, (e) Radiologist.

15. What physician is trained to take care of the mentally ill? (a) Psychologist, (b) *Psychiatrist*, (c) Neurologist, (d) Osteopath, (e) Obstetrician.

16. What physician delivers babies and takes care of the pregnant patient during the prenatal period? (a) Pediatrician, (b)*Obstetrician*, (c) Gynecologist, (d) Urologist, (e) Dermatologist.

17. What physician cares for infants and children up to the age of puberty? (a) *Pediatrician*, (b) Obstetrician, (c) Gynecologist, (d) Radiologist, (e) Neurologist.

18. What physician treats disorders of the female reproductive organs? (a) Internist, (b) Urologist, (c) Obstetrician, (d) *Gynecologist*, (e) Orthopedist.

19. State medicine differs from socialized medicine most in: (a) Total cost, (b) The plan of professional education, (c) Equipment provided to physicians, (d) *The extent of governmental control*, (e) The agency which operates the plan.

20. The first federal consumer legislation was enacted by Congress in 1906. It dealt with control over: (a)*Food and drugs*, (b) Drugs only, (c) Foods, drugs, and cosmetics, (d) Drugs and therapeutic devices, (e) Foods only.

## Matching Items

1. Treats disease of the stomach and intestines (k)
2. Treats such conditions as asthma, hay fever, allergies (m)
3. Is not a medical doctor, trained to examine the eyes for glasses, not trained to treat diseases of the eye (m)
4. Treats ailments of the ears, throat, sinuses, and nose (m)
5. Specializes in diseases of the bones and joints (f)
6. Is a doctor trained to care for the mentally ill (i)
7. Delivers babies and cares for pregnant mother (a)
8. Treats infants and children up to puberty (b)
9. Specializes in performing operations (m)
10. Is expert in diagnosis and treatment of medical conditions of the entire body (c)
11. Specializes in treating kidney conditions and male genital disorders (e)
12. Specializes in interpreting X-rays (l)

a. Obstetrician
b. Pediatrician
c. Internist
d. Gynecologist
e. Urologist
f. Orthopedist
g. Ophthalmologist
h. Dermatologist
i. Psychiatrist
j. Neurologist
k. Gastroenterologist
l. Radiologist
m. None of these

## Essay Items

1. Identify criteria that might help in evaluating the reliability of health information.

2. The modern consumer is afforded some protection through legislation that has been passed at the federal level. Identify recent major laws that provide protection for the health consumer, and briefly discuss their basic provisions.

3. List some of the signs or characteristics whereby an individual might be able to detect medical quackery or the quack.

4. One of the most vital factors in promoting and maintaining healthful living is choosing health advisors. State the criteria and practical guidelines that you might use in the selection of a competent personal physician were you to change your permanent residence.

5. State and discuss several important principles to be considered in the purchase of a health insurance policy.

6. Identify some of the major national agencies and organizations that help provide protection for the health consumer. Briefly discuss the role, functions, and basic responsibilities of each.

7. Discuss the current issues in the controversy over national health insurance plans and care.

# HEALTH MAINTENANCE

*Part Two* ❧ *Chapter* 7

---

## BEHAVIORAL OBJECTIVES

The Student

- plots the basic structure of the human organism and the general body plan

- compares the different systems of the body as to structure and function

- predicts the influence of different endocrine secretions on basic bodily functions

- synthesizes the relationship between mind and body and the importance of such interrelationship

- identifies the mechanisms by which vision and hearing take place and the function of the teeth and skin

- practices the measures that help to prevent and reduce malfunction of the body

## SUPPLEMENTARY TEACHING AIDS

### Films

*Code Blue*, color, 27½ min. There is an ever-growing need for minority representation in every field of health. This film lists reasons why blacks and other minority groups should consider careers in medicine or allied health. A hit with all youth groups because "it tells it like it is." Modern Talking Pictures, 3 East 54th Street, New York, N. Y. 10022.

*Diabetics Unknown*, The film presents medical and background information and case histories. Diabetics describe how they discovered they had diabetes, what they are doing about it, and how it affects their lives. Public Affairs Film Library, 267 W. 25th St., New York, N. Y. 10001.

*Doorway to Dental Health*, color, 14½ min. A unique, entertaining motion picture featuring Doctor Prevent, a dentist who guides a young patient on a tour of his office, demonstrates proper brushing and flossing techniques, and informs the viewer of the need for regular dental checkups and good diet. Modern Talking Pictures, 3 East 54th Street, New York, N. Y. 10022.

*Fluoridation: A White Paper*, color, 13 min. The relationship between fluoridation in the community water supply and good dental health is discussed by dentists, scientists, an engineer, and a lawyer. Modern Talking Pictures, 3 East 54th Street, New York, N. Y. 10022.

*Gateway to Health*, color, 20 min. Simple rules of dental care and good health are presented in a factual story by a group of children and adults. Supervision of dental care by a personal dentist through regular checkups is recommended. Association-Sterling Films, 600 Grand Avenue, Ridgefield, N. J. 07657.

*The Hospital, the Surgeon, and You*, color, 14 min. This film offers a look at behind-the-scenes activities of hospital life, and surgical procedures in particular. The education and training of surgeons is discussed in detail. Modern Talking Pictures, 3 East 54th Street, New York, N. Y. 10022.

*House of Man: Respiration in Man*, color, 26 min. This film describes the structure and function of the respiratory system and demonstrates modern techniques of clinical diagnosis and the relationship of air pollution to the respiratory system physiology. Encyclopedia Britannica, Education Corp., 425 N. Michigan Ave., Chicago, Ill. 60611.

*Preventive Dentistry in B Sharp*, color, 14 min. An eminent composer (played by Avery Schreiber) dedicates a symphony to preventive dentistry in this humorous yet informative film. Basic facts about cleaning and maintaining healthy teeth and gums are related. Modern Talking Pictures, 3 East 54th Street, New York, N. Y. 10022.

*Stress*, b-w, 11 min. Dr. Selye defines stress and its relationship to body systems, particularly pituitary and adrenal glands. Contemporary Films, McGraw-Hill, 828 Custer Ave., Evanston, Ill. 60203.

*Teeth ... Are Good Things to Have*, color, 13½ min. Plaque— everyone is talking about it, and now this film musically tells the story. Emphasis is on P.D. (Preventive Dentistry), and this light, amusing, animated message shows how a few minutes of dental care at home each day can prevent pain and save money. Association-Sterling Films, 600 Grand Avenue, Ridgefield, N. J. 07657.

*To Conserve and Protect*, color, 14½ min. Narrator James Mason explores the aspects of noise pollution, its causes, deleterious effects on human beings, and what can be done to conserve and protect the hearing ability. The first part is factual; the second part is a staged dramatic community example. Modern Talking Pictures, 2322 New Hyde Park Rd., New Hyde Park, N. Y. 11040.

Write for Catalog: National Society for the Prevention of Blindness, 79 Madison Ave., New York, N. Y. 10016.

Transparency Originals (See Part 3 of Handbook)

## ORGANIZATIONS THAT HAVE MATERIALS *

Allergy Foundation of America, 801 Second Ave., New York, N. Y. 10017.

American Association of Ophthalmology, 1100 Seventeenth St., N. W., Washington, D. C. 20036.

American Dental Association, Bureau of Dental Health Education, 22 East Superior St., Chicago, Ill. 60611.

American Foundation for the Blind, Inc., 15 West Sixteenth St., New York, N. Y. 10011.

American Hospital Association, 840 North Lake Shore Dr., Chicago, Ill. 60611.

American Medical Association, Bureau of Health Education, 535 North Dearborn St., Chicago, Ill. 60610.

American Occupational Therapy Association, 600 Executive Blvd., Suite 200, Rockville, Md. 20852.

American Optometric Association, Public Information Division, 7000 Chippewa St., St. Louis, Mo. 63119.

American Podiatry Association, Council on Education, 20 Chevy Chase Circle, N. W., Washington, D. C. 22015.

American Speech and Hearing Association, 1001 Connecticut Ave., Washington, D. C. 20006.

Better Vision Institute, 230 Park Ave., New York, N. Y. 10017.

Council for Exceptional Children, Suite 900, 1411 Jefferson Davis Highway, Arlington, Va. 22202.

Department of Health, Education and Welfare, Public Health Service, 5600 Fishers Lane, Rockville, Md. 20852.

Metropolitan Life Insurance Company, 1 Madison Avenue, New York, N. Y. 10010.

National Institute of Allergy and Infectious Diseases, Office of Information, Bethesda, Md. 20014.

National Recreation and Park Association, 1601 North Kent St., Arlington, Va. 22209.

National Society for the Prevention of Blindness, Inc., 79 Madison Ave., New York, N. Y. 10016.

*The addresses of these organizations and their policies concerning the sending of materials are subject to change without notice.*

## STUDENT INVOLVEMENT
### Investigations

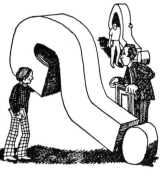

Identify ways in which the body's specialized organs and systems work together in performing complex actions and in meeting stresses of the environment.

What are some of the relationships that exist between the endocrines, the emotions, and body functions?

Compile a list of the functions performed by various body systems. What diseases are produced by malfunction or disturbance?

Compare views of health in various philosophical and religious groups. Examples: Christian Science, Zen, Theosophy, Yoga.

Report on various beliefs and dietary regulations of different religions.

What are the phenomena involved in "Faith Healing"?

What is the relationship of mind and body according to the system of Yoga?

Should the cost of dental care be included in health insurance policies?

Are local community water supplies fluoridated? What action was instigated to bring this about, or what activities are presently directed toward instituting fluoridation? Why is this such a hot issue in some communities?

What ways can a person with a hearing deficiency make maximal use of his environment (room arrangement, seating, noise levels)?

Is there a rational basis for prescribing glasses for a student with normal vision?

What are the methods of testing vision? What are the limitations of each method?

Investigate special classes and facilities for children with learning problems related to poor vision or hearing. What arrangements are being made to accommodate "rubella babies" with hearing or vision disability who were born during the 1963-64 epidemic? Are the local schools equipped to handle the problems of these children?

### Action

Perform laboratory tests to determine effectiveness of popularly advertised mouth washes.

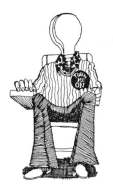

How valuable are the vision and screening tests in elementary schools? Compare number and type of disabilities detected in various sections of the community. Also, how many case referrals are actually followed up with proper treatment?

Collect old eyeglass frames and deliver them to the local Lions Club for their vision program, or send them to New Eyes for the Needy, Morristown, N.J.

Take soundings; meter the decibel level at local rock dances. Do you believe listening to loud rock music over a period of time can impair hearing?

Compare the costs for eye checkups among various professionals: ophthalmologists and optometrists. Compare costs for lenses and frames.

Make an appointment for that health examination or dental checkup that has been put off for some time now.

Visit studios and "health clubs" that offer courses in mind-body exercises. Report observations.

Classify yourself on the basis of Shelton's body type system. How has your body type influenced your skill in various activities?

## BASIC SOURCE MATERIALS

Bernhardt, Mary, and Bob Sprague, "Are We Depriving Our Children of Healthy Teeth?" *Family Health*, 9:29-33, April, 1977.

Campbell, Agnes, "Subjective Measures of Well-Being," *American Psychologist*, 31:117-24, February, 1976.

Chien, Agnes, and Lawrence Schneiderman, "A Comparison of Health Care Utilization by Husbands and Wives," *Journal of Current Health*, 1:118-26, Winter, 1975.

"Coping with Stress Effectively," *Intellect*, 106:13-14, July, 1977.

Crawford, Robert, "You Are Dangerous to Your Health," *Social Policy*, 8:10-20, January-February, 1978.

Gastrin, Gisela, "How Education Helps," *World Health*, 14-17, November, 1975.

Kahn, Carol, "Do You Dream (Perchance) of Sleeping?" *Family Health*, 9:36-39, 57, September, 1977.

Kennedy, Alan, "New Family Practice Specialists," *Medical World News*, 16:65-78, October, 1975.

Kirscht, John P., "Public Response to Various Written Appeals to Participate in Health Screening," *Public Health Reports*, 90:539-543, November-December, 1975.

Kosidlak, Janet, "Improving Health Care for Troubled Youths," *American Journal of Nursing*, 76:95-97, January, 1976.

Levin, Lowell S., "Self-Care and Health Planning," *Social Policy*, 8:47-54, November-December, 1978.

Mayer, Jean, "Build Yourself a Better Heart", *Family Health*, 8:34-39, February, 1976.

Moen, Elizabeth, "The Reluctance of the Elderly to Accept Help," *Social Problems*, 25:293-303, February, 1978.

Mortensen, Barbara B., "Dental Myths and Misconceptions," *Family Health*, 9:14, December, 1977.

O'Donnell, Walter, "Who's Guilty of Overhospitalization? Me and Probably You," *Medical Economics*, 52:80-85, October 13, 1975.

Oppenheim, Irene, "Third-Part Payments," *Social Policy*, 8:55-58, November-December, 1977.

Roman, Stanford A., "Health Maintenance Organizations — Are They for the Inner Cities?" *Journal of Community Health*, 1:127-31, Winter, 1975.

Runninger, Jack, "Are You Seeing as Well as You Should? Test Your Eye-Q," *Family Health*, 8:30-31, January, 1976.

Sehnent, Keith, "The Activated Patient," *Family Health*, 8:14-15, February, 1976.

Starr, Paul, "The Undelivered Health System," *The Public Internist*, 42:66-85, Winter, 1976.

Trubo, Richard, "When Your Dreams Turn into Nightmares," *Family Health*, 8:40-43, 74, 76, March, 1976.

Walker, Sydney, "Blood Sugar and Emotional Storms: Sugar Doctors Push Hypoglycemia," *Psychology Today*, 9:69-74, July, 1975.

Weber, Melva, "Acne — Myths and Facts," *Family Health*, 7:43-45, August, 1975.

Williams, Gurney, "Your Aching Back — And What You Can Do about It," *Family Health*, 9:26-31, March, 1977.

Wilston, Barbara, "How I Tried to Navigate the Health System... and Didn't Succeed," *Social Policy*, 8:59-65, November-December, 1977.

Wycoff, Samuel, "Current Concepts in Preventive Dentistry," *The American College Health Association Journal*, 23:356-58, June, 1975.

Zizmor, Jonathan, and John Foreman, "Understanding Skin Care," *Family Health*, 9:28-29, May, 1977.

## TEST QUESTIONS

### Multiple Choice Items

1. The recommended way to prevent athlete's foot is to: (a) Avoid bathing in a public place, (b) *Carefully wash and dry the feet daily*, (c) Use fungicide powders on the feet each day, (d) Avoid the use of rubber-soled shoes, (e) Use a footbath.

2. What color lens is best to avoid when purchasing sun glasses? (a) Gray, (b) Green, (c) Blue, (d) Tan, (e) *Brown*.

3. Myopic vision means: (a) Farsightedness, (b) *Nearsightedness*, (c) Astigmatism, (d) Strabismus, (e) Presbyopia.

4. Glaucoma occurs most frequently: (a) *In women after 35 years of age,* (b) In men after 35 years of age, (c) In young women, (d) In children, (e) In infants.

5. Which specialist does not treat the eyes? (a) The Optician, (b) Ophthalmologist, (c) Oculist, (d) *Otologist,* (e) Ophthalmic optician.

6. Cataract is: (a) A growth over the front of the eye, (b) A thickening of the cornea, (c) Hemorrhage of the retina, (d) *An opacity of the lens,* (e) A degeneration of the optic nerve.

7. Which of the following is not a visual abnormality? (a) Amblyopia, (b) Myopia, (c) Astigmatism, (d) *Ménière's disease,* (e) Strabismus.

8. A cause of deafness that cannot be alleviated is: (a) Otosclerosis, (b) *Nerve type,* (c) Middle ear infection, (d) Drug sensitivity, (e) Otitis media.

9. The best lighting for doing near point tasks is: (a) Spotlight directly pinpointed on the task, (b) Light from over the right shoulder, (c) *Well lighted room by diffused or indirect lights,* (d) Daylight in preference to artificial lighting, (e) None of the above.

10. Gingivitis is a disease of the : (a) Nasal sinuses, (b) Tongue, (c) Dental pulp, (d) *Gums,* (e) Epidermis.

11. Reading in poor light or in an uncomfortable position usually results in: (a) Farsightedness, (b) Damage to the eyes, (c) Styes and inflammation, (d) *General fatigue,* (e) Nearsightedness.

12. The sensitive cells of the eye that help to receive light stimuli in image formation are the: (a) *Retina,* (b) Cornea, (c) Lenses, (d) Stopes, (e) Cochlea.

13. The "master gland," the size of a pea, is located in the brain and secretes several hormones that influence growth, metabolism, and sex development in the male and female. It is the: (a) *Pituitary,* (b) Adrenal, (c) Pancreas, (d) Thyroid, (e) Ovaries and testes.

14. Masses, or groups, of cells of particular types are called: (a) *Tissues,* (b) Organs, (c) Cytoplasms, (d) Nuclei, (e) Cells.

15. The soft organs of the body are termed: (a) Systems, (b) *Viscera*, (c) Tissues, (d) Ligaments, (e) Hematopoietics.

16. Dwarfism, Acromegaly, and Giantism are three conditions caused by a glandular malfunction of the (a) Thymus gland, (b) Adrenal gland, (c) *Pituitary gland*, (d) Parathyroid gland, (e) Thyroid gland.

17. A dentist who specializes in treating gum disease in adults is: (a) an orthodontist, (b) a pediatrician, (c) *a periodontist*, (d) an endodontist.

18. Brushing the teeth: (a) Once a day is as good as brushing more often, (b) *Will reduce but not completely prevent tooth decay*, (c) Will prevent tooth decay completely if the right toothpaste is used, (d) Is most effective when the brush moves forward and backward across the teeth, (e) Should be started at about the age the child enters school.

19. Which is not a myth about teeth: (a) A slightly chipped tooth can be ignored, (b) An abscessed tooth must be extracted, (c) Bad teeth are inherited, (d) *Dental caries are about as common as the common cold*, (e) Perfect deciduous teeth mean perfect permanent teeth.

20. Which of the following statements is most correct concerning occlusion? It means: (a) When each tooth touches those beside it, (b) *The relationship between the upper and lower teeth*, (c) Usually perfect, (d) The same for all persons, (e) Different in men than in women.

## Matching Items

1. Farsightedness (f)
2. Middle ear infection (i)
3. Trench mouth (h)
4. Equilibrium (e)
5. Emotional shock (b)
6. Hearing difficulty (a)
7. Oculist (d)
8. Cretinism (j)
9. Noise level (g)
10. Irregular curvature of the lens (c)

a. Presbycusis
b. Psychogenic disorder
c. Astigmatism
d. Ophthalmologist
e. Homeostasis
f. Hyperopia
g. Decibel
h. Vincent's Infection
i. Otitis Media
j. Thyroid
k. None of these

## Essay Items

1. List good habits to develop when using eyes in artificial light.

2. What essential activities should be stressed when planning a program of prevention of hearing loss.

3. List at least six functions of the skin.

4. In what ways can emotions affect well-being? Provide concrete examples of these influences.

5. List and describe the different sensory receptors of the body.

6. Discuss various types of noise pollution and what actions may be taken to stop the deleterious effects.

7. The endocrine system exerts a profound influence on all body functions. Illustrate some of the more important of these influences by specific examples.

8. Discuss what is meant by the famous statement "A sound mind in a sound body."

9. What are the implications of less restricted advertisement of services provided by eye specialists?

# FITNESS FOR LIVING

*Part Two* ❧ *Chapter 8*

---

**BEHAVIORAL OBJECTIVES**

The Student:

● defines physical fitness in relation to the concept of total fitness

● describes the characteristics of the fit individual

● predicts the effect of exercise on cardiovascular efficiency, body function, and health

● lists some of the effects of fatigue in relation to health and efficiency

● evaluates the importance of sleep, rest, relaxation, recreation, posture, and proper body mechanics in the maintenance of well-being

● Illustrates the more significant structural and foot defects that interfere with optimal health

# SUPPLEMENTARY TEACHING AIDS

Contact your local chapter of the American Heart Association. Transparency Originals (See Part 3 of Handbook)

---

## STUDENT INVOLVEMENT

### Investigations

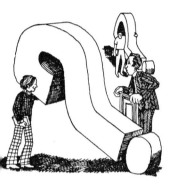

Identify ways in which the health hazards of modern living differ from those in the early days of the United States. What factors have been most responsible for these changes, and how do they relate to fitness?

Compile a list of the activities in which you regularly participate. Compare these to recommendations for adequate exercise made by Cooper in *New Aerobics.*

Why are sufficient sleep, rest, relaxation, and exercise necessities for the maintenance of fitness?

Indicate some of the major points to consider in the selection of physical activities. Include factors to be avoided in such choices as well as those to be recommended.

Define fatigue and describe the chemistry of the process. What are the physiological and psychological effects of fatigue on the body?

List some of the conditions of the environment that help to enhance sleep. Describe the physiological and psychological effects of sleep deprivation. What are negative long-term side effects of dependence on sleeping pills or sleep aids?

Compute during a week's time the average length of time spent per day in vigorous exercises, rest, relaxation, sleep, and recreation. Why or why not are these amounts adequate for you?

What effect do stimulants have on the body (for example, No-Doz, and amphetamines)? Are they safe for athletes? Is it illegal and unethical to use drugs in athletics?

# Action

Conduct a survey of members of all ages at a health club. Determine attitudes, motivation, and health habits. Why have these people joined a health club? What benefits do they receive?

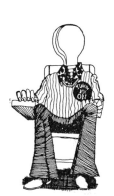

Conduct your own personal fitness test. Outline an exercise program. Then STICK WITH IT.

Join a swim, tennis, hiking, or bicycle club. Report on your fitness level.

Survey recreational facilities available in your community. Are they adequate? How might they be improved? Are facilities available for the elderly? Send observations to park and recreation bureau.

Visit local high schools. What program is there for fitness and personal development within the regular required Physical Education program?

Visit a home for the elderly to learn what sport or recreational activities are available and utilized. How valuable is recreation to the aging?

## BASIC SOURCE MATERIALS

Ashby, Neal, "How the Famous Stay Fit," *Family Health*, 8:45-46, April, 1976.

Barreto, Delia M., *The Muscles: A Study Aid for Allied Health Professional Students*, Flushing, N.Y.: Scholium International, Inc., 1974.

Bowerman, William J. et al., *Jogging*, New York: Grosset & Dunlap, 1976.

Cooper, Kenneth, *Aerobics for Women*, Philadelphia: Lippincott, 1972.

Darden, Ellington, *Nutrition and Athletic Performance*, Pasadena, Calif.: The Athletic Press, 1976.

Franco, Marjorie, "Don't Aim for the All-Stars—Just Hit the Ball," *Today's Health*, 53:45-48, September, 1975.

"Hard Work Vs. Heart Attack," *Science Digest*, 77:28-29, June, 1975.

Holland, George J., and Elwood Craig Davis, *Values of Physical Activity*, 3rd ed., Dubuque, Iowa: William C. Brown Company, 1975.

Katch, Frank I., and William D. McArdle, *Nutrition, Weight Control and Exercise*, Boston: Houghton Mifflin Company, 1977.

Kaye, Elizabeth, "Is All This Muscle That Healthy?" *Family Health*, 9:20-24, December, 1977.

Krizan, Thomas, "The Busiest Room in the School," *Journal of Physical Education and Recreation*, 47:33-34, February, 1976.

Macey, Robert I., *Human Physiology*, Englewood Cliffs, N. J.: Prentice-Hall, 1975.

Mathews, Donald K., and Edward L. Fox, *The Physiology Basis of Physical Education and Athletes*, Philadelphia: W.B. Saunders Company, 1976.

McElroy, William D., and Swanson, Carl P., *Music Physiology*, Englewood Cliffs, N.J.: Prentice-Hall, 1974.

Morehouse, Laurence E., and Leonard Gross, "Shape Up," *Family Health*, 7:34-37, 66-67, February, 1975.

Osman, Jack, *Thin from Within*, New York: Hart Publishing Company, 1976.

Rhodes, Russell, L., *Man at His Best*, New York: Doubleday and Company, 1974.

Sharkey, Brian J., *Physiology and Physical Activity*, New York: Harper and Row, Publishers, 1975.

Smith, Nathan J., *Food for Sport*, Palo Alto, Calif.: Bull Publishing Company, 1976.

Snyder, Eldon E., and Joseph E. Kevlin, "Women Athletes and Aspects of Psychological Well-Being and Body Image," *Research Quarterly*, 46:191-99, May, 1975.

Spackman, Robert R., "Easy Isometrics," *Family Health*, 9:48-51, May, 1977.

Wilkinson, Bud., "Our Guide to the Best Sports for Your Health," *Today's Health*, 50:16-21, 65-67, May, 1972.

## TEST QUESTIONS

### Multiple Choice Items

1. Total fitness is a combination of the same basic components that are implied by: (a) *Health,* (b) Athletic ability, (c) Age, (d) Skill, (e) Emotional stability.

2. Physical fitness is the capacity to do: (a) A job, (b) *Work,* (c) An exercise, (d) A problem, (e) Strenuous activity.

3. A planned program of physical activity is essential today because of: (a) The increased size of man's stature, (b) The availability of more gymnasia, (c) *Complex living which limits natural muscular activity,* (d) Dense urban population, (e) Rich diets.

4. Most authorities agree that college-age adults require: (a) Light exercise, (b) Infrequent exercise, (c) *Vigorous exercise,* (d) No planned exercise, (e) Primarily individual sports.

5. Which of the following is *not* an accepted principle of exercise: (a) Coronary artery disease demands both a preventive approach and a therapeutic approach, (b)

Physical training lowers the resting heart rate, (c) Surveys from many countries indicate that active people have less coronary artery disease, (d) *Exercise does not play an important role in the lipid deposit theory of arteriosclerosis,* (e) Exercise is becoming a vital part of the convalescent treatment of heart patients.

6. The most important way in which exercise contributes to the health of the body is through: (a) *Stimulating the circulation of the blood,* (b) Increasing the number of muscles, (c) Eliminating ulcers, (d) Increasing the strength of the bones.

7. The most important single factor in the attainment of physical fitness is: (a) Diet, (b) Sleep and rest, (c) Recreation, (d) Freedom from worry, (e) *Exercise.*

8. A forward curvature of the lumbar region of the back that results in an anteroposterior deviation called "hollow back" is termed: (a) Kyphosis, (b) Inversion, (c) Scoliosis, (d) *Lordosis,* (e) Metamorphosis.

9. The most popular leisure time, if measured by money spent, is: (a) Reading, (b) Movies, (c) Magazine reading, (d) Boating, (e) *Fishing.*

10. Exercise may play a role in the prevention of death from coronary artery diseases because: (a) *It hastens the clearance of fat from the blood,* (b) It activates the system that destroys normal blood clotting substances, (c) It increases the coronary collateral circulation, (d) All of the above, (e) None of the above.

11. Physically fit persons: (a) Work with greater efficiency, (b) Require less energy to complete a given task, (c) Recover more quickly from fatigue, (d) *All of the above,* (e) None of the above.

12. An exercise plan to be effective must be based on two important principles. These are: (a) The body must perform at its present capacity weekly and the body must be taxed beyond its normal capacity to develop, (b) The body must perform at its present capacity daily and the body must not be taxed beyond its normal capacity, (c) *The body must perform at its present capacity daily, and the body must be taxed beyond its normal capacity in order to develop,* (d) Periodically, the body may be required to perform beyond its normal capacity and minimal stress must be applied, (e) The body must be required

to perform at its capacity and never beyond normal capacity.

13. In choosing an activity that will increase longevity and promote general fitness, particularly endurance, the activity should: (a) Build muscles, (b) Build flexibility, (c) *Stimulate the cardiovascular and respiratory systems*, (d) Increase strength, (d) Develop agility.

14. Scientific evidence suggests that some vigorous exercise daily: (a) Decreases metabolic functioning, (b) Increases inelasticity of the coronary arteries, (c) Appreciably increases caloric needs, (d) *Increases organic vigor*, (e) Increases cholesterol levels.

15. The most common cause of fatigue among college students is: (a) Pathological in origin, (b) Muscular in origin, (c) Physiological in origin, (d) *Emotional in origin*, (e) Social in origin.

16. Relaxation is necessary to reduce everyday tension. The most efficient way to accomplish relaxation is to provide for: (a) A daily nap, (b) *A change of pace several times during the day*, (c) A long vacation at least once every year, (d) Ten-minute rest periods every one or two hours, (e) Adequate periods of sleep.

17. Isometric exercises (a) Are not performed in an immovable object, (b) Are not self-resistive exercises, (c) *Do not contribute to stamina and endurance*, (d) Do not develop specific groups of muscles, (e) Are not based on muscle contractions.

18. Motivation for keeping fit in the world today probably: (a) Stems from the demands of modern society, (b) Is unnecessary except in times of national crisis, (c) *Must be generated by the individual himself*, (d) Is now being supplied by the governmental stress on physical fitness, (e) Is incompatible with the stress on mechanization.

19. The type and amount of exercise taken should be selected according to: (a) The size of the person, (b) The availability of the activity, (c) The cost of the activity, (d) One's capacity, (e) *All of these*.

20. The amount of sleep needed is: (a) The same for all persons, (b) The same for the same person at all ages, (c)

Greater for light eaters than for heavy eaters, (d) *Influenced by the amount of nervous and muscular fatigue,* (e) Not related to working efficiency.

## Matching Items

1. Deterioration of efficiency (f)
2. Ninety percent of all Americans (e)
3. Cardiovascular disease (g)
4. Medical supervision (i)
5. Movement (a)
6. Humpback (d)
7. Arthritis (c)
8. Decrease in metabolic processes (j)
9. Lateral curvature of spine (b)
10. Longitudinal arch (h)

a. Isotonics
b. Scoliosis
c. Postural defects
d. Kyphosis
e. Recreation
f. Fatigue
g. Lack of exercise
h. Flat feet
i. Sleeping pills
j. Sleep

## Essay Items

1. In what ways does life in the United States today differ from that of only two generations ago? What effect have such changes had on the quality of life and general fitness of the population?

2. Discuss some of the specific effects of physical activity on the various systems of the body.

3. Briefly describe the general chemistry of the fatigue process. Include some of the psychological, as well as physiological, effects of fatigue on the body.

4. List some of the conditions that help to enhance sleep, and indicate factors that may prevent it.

5. Why are rest, sleep, relaxation, recreation, and exercise important essentials in the maintenance of sound health?

6. Situation: You are an elementary teacher. A fellow teacher wants to have all the students go through a rigorous exercise program at lunch time, the last fifteen minutes of the lunch period, on a daily basis. He has asked you to help convince the principal that this is a "good and necessary" program. What are some things that you might have to consider before you decide whether to support this program?

# THE SCIENCE OF NUTRITION

*Part Two* 🐂 *Chapter* **9**

## BEHAVIORAL OBJECTIVES

The Student

- believes that what one eats has a direct influence on what one is

- applies the principles of the science of nutrition to personal dietary habits

- evaluates critically the mass of information and misinformation propounded about foods and nutrients

- selects a diet that will maintain weight within normal ranges

- prevents the acquisition of food-borne diseases by proper preparation and storage of food

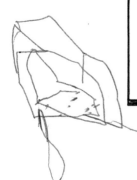

# SUPPLEMENTARY TEACHING AIDS

## Films

*Eat to Your Heart's Content*, color, 12½ min. This film hits the high spots of the importance of diet, emphasizing how saturated fats, high cholesterol and lack of exercise set the stage for heart attack. It explains how a lifetime diet can be easy and fun with the right selection of foods. American Heart Association, Film Library, 267 West 25th St., New York, N. Y. 10001.

*Hunger in America*, b-w, 58 min. 1968. A grim and factual picture of ten million Americans for whom this film is reality. This is a graphic demonstration of the need for America to reassess its Federal programs that provide lard and peanut butter to people desperate for fruit, fresh milk and meat. C.B.S., Education and Publishing Dept., 383 Madison Ave., New York, N. Y. 10017.

*Jenny is a Good Thing*, color, 18 min. This film dramatically shows that the nutrition program plays a major role and is an integral part of the daily activities in a quality Head Start Center. Narrated by Burt Lancaster. Leader's Discussion Guide upon request. Modern Talking Pictures, 160 E. Grand Ave., Chicago, Ill. 60611.

*Read the Label—Set a Better Table*, color, 14 min. This film demonstrates the value of reading food labels to determine the most nutritious buy for one's money. Most food packages now list the nutrients and the percentage of U.S. Recommended Daily Allowance contained in the product. A dynamic film that is a must for all nutrition education classes. Features Dick Van Dyke. Modern Talking Pictures, 3 East 54th Street, New York, N. Y. 10022.

*The Tenement*, b-w, 40 min. 1967. Tenants of a Chicago slum home reveal the despair and the futility of their lives and express hope that their children will be able to escape the trap of poverty. C.B.S., Education and Publishing Dept., 383 Madison Ave., New York, N. Y. 10017.

*Three Times a Day*, color, 25 min. Who would have thought that the chubby, overfed baby would foster poor eating habits throughout his life? This film demonstrates the relationship between daily diet and heart disease. *Three Times a Day* offers sound advice on how to establish a good diet. Association—Sterling Films, 600 Grand Avenue, Ridgefield, N. J. 07657.

*Toward the Victory of Health*, color, 14½ min. A captivating account of the conquest of nutritional deficiencies, bringing to the fore dietary research and the science of nutrition. Note: The first half of this film is an excellent historical presentation, while the second half is commercial and limited in its use. Modern Talking Pictures, 2323 New Hyde Park Rd., New Hyde Park, N. Y. 11040.

*The Waistland*, color, 27 min. Losing weight is serious business. This TOPS Club, Inc. (Take Off Pounds Sensibly) film explains how the organization bases a highly successful weight reduction program on sensible eating habits throughout one's lifetime. Diet myths and fads are exposed and viewers are enlightened as to the causes and cures for overweight. Association—Sterling FIlms, 600 Grand Avenue, Ridgefield, N. J. 07657.

Transparency Originals (See Part 3 of Handbook)

### Filmstrip

*Food and Nutrution*. Five color filmstrips, cassettes or record. Content of this set includes prenatal nutrition, nutritional needs of young children, and the relationship of nutritional deficiencies to physical and mental disability. Parents' Magazine Films, Inc., 52 Vanderbilt Ave., New York, N. Y. 10017.

## ORGANIZATIONS THAT HAVE
## MATERIALS *

American Dairy Association, 20 North Wacker Drive, Chicago, Ill. 60606.

American Diabetes Association, Inc., 18 East 48th St., New York, N. Y. 10017.

American Dietetic Association, 620 N. Michigan Ave., Chicago, Ill. 60611.

American Dry Milk Institute, Inc., 130 North Franklin St., Chicago, Ill. 60606.

American Home Economics Association, 2010 Massachusetts Ave., N. W., Washington, D. C. 20036.

American School Food Service Association, P. O. Box 8811, Denver, Co., 80210.

Carnation Milk Company, Homes Service Department, 5045 Wilshire Blvd., Los Angeles, Calif. 90036.

Cereal Institute, Inc., 135 South LaSalle Street, Chicago, Ill. 60603.

Florida Citrus Commission, Production Department, Lakeland, Fla. 33802.

Food and Drug Administration, Department of Health, Education and Welfare, Washington, D. C. 20025.

General Mills, Public Relations Department, 9200 Wazata Blvd., Minneapolis, Minn. 55413.

Kellogg Company, Public Affairs Department, 235 Porter St., Battle Creek, Mich. 49016.

National Dairy Council, 111 North Canal St., Chicago, Ill. 60606.

National Livestock and Meat Board, 407 S. Dearborn St., Chicago, Ill. 60605.

Nutrition Foundation, Inc., 99 Park Ave., New York, N. Y. 10016.

Pet Milk Company, Director of Home Economics, 1401 Arcade Building, St. Louis, Mo. 63111.

Ralston Purina Company, Checkerboard Square, St. Louis, Mo. 63102.

*The addresses of these organizations and their policies concerning the sending of materials are subject to change without notice.

## STUDENT INVOLVEMENT

### Investigations

Compute personal average daily caloric needs. Relate these to optimum daily requirements.

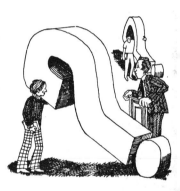

Plan a diet using the four basic foods that will facilitate the loss of two pounds per week, exercise being held constant.

Defend or refute the statement that "formula diet foods" are good to use in a weight reduction diet.

Survey the cereal section in a supermarket to find the cereals, both dried and cooked, that are the most nutritious.

Compare prices in the average market with those in a health food store.

Display "fad" foods or "health foods." Explain the contents, the food value and the attraction of these foods to certain people.

Plan a menu without meat. Substitute other foods high in protein to meet the daily adult requirements. Compare this cost with a meat-meal.

### Action

Prepare a "Natural Foods" meal. Invite your friends and your professor. Have a "freak-out" on Food.

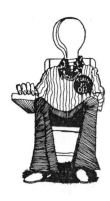

Visit a local supermarket. Report back on its consumer education program.

Conduct a survey among the elderly with limited incomes. Volunteer to assist in obtaining Food Stamps, with shopping, or serving in a senior citizens' hot meal program.

Plan your personal weight control program. Report on success or failure.

Read several copies of *Prevention* magazine, Emmaus, Pa. 18049. Analyze articles for "truthfulness." Report on Food Cults to class.

## BASIC SOURCE MATERIALS

Annis, L. F., *The Child before Birth*, New York: Cornell University Press, 1978.

Becher, Marshall, H. et al., "The Health Belief Model and Prediction of Dietary Compliance," *Journal of Health and Social Behavior*, 18:348-65, December, 1977.

Bogan, Kathy A., "Nutrition and Mental Health: What Is the Relationship?" *Occupational Health Nursing*, 24:17-20, February, 1976.

Breeling, James L., "Are We Snacking Our Way to Malnutrition," *Today's Health*, 48:48-51, January, 1970.

Breneman, J. C., *Basics of Food Allergy*, Springfield, Illinois: Charles C. Thomas, Bannerstone House, 1978.

Calvert, Gene Paul, "Intellectual Convictions of Health Food Consumers," *Journal of Nutrition Education*, 7:95-98, July-September, 1975.

Committee on Nutrition of Mother and Preschool Child, "Fetal and Infant Nutrition and Susceptibility to Obesity," Summary of Workshop, *Nutrition Reviews*, 36:122-26, April, 1978.

Deutsch, Ronald M., *The Family Guide to Better Food and Better Health*, Des Moines, Iowa: Meredith Corporation, 1971.

Fisch, R., et al., "Obesity and Leanness at Birth and Their Relationship to Body Habitus in Later Childhood," *Pediatrics*, 56:521-28, October, 1975.

Goldberg, Jeanne, "Vegetarianism," *Family Health*, 10:30-31, April, 1978.

Lewin, Rober, "Starved Brains," *Psychology Today*, 9:29-33, September, 1975.

Loxson, Rosalino, "Changing Obesity Patterns," *Nursing Outlook*, 23:711-13, November, 1975.

Matthews, Ruth H., and Martha Y. Workman, "Nutrient Content of Selected Bag Foods," *Journal of the American Dietetic Association*, 72:27-30, January, 1978.

Mayer, Jean, "Give Thanks for Safe Food," *Family Health*, 9:37, November, 1977.

Poolton, Martha A., "What Can We Do about Food Habits?" *Journal of School Health*, 48:646-48, January, 1978.

Rae, Jessie, and Burke, Anne Louise, "Counselling the Elderly on Nutrition in a Community Health Care System," *Journal of the American Geriatrics Society*, 25:130-135, March, 1978.

Smith, Elizabeth B., "A Guide To Good Eating the Vegetarian Way," *Journal of Nutrition Education*, 7:109-11, July-September, 1975.

"There's A Fly In The Milk Bottle," *Medical World News*, 15:30-34, May 17, 1974.

Vinson, Leonard, "Modifying The American Diet To Stem The Tide of Coronary Heart Disease," *Nursing Care*, 8:8-13, November, 1975.

Weatherholtz, Willard, and Michele Bremer, "Nutrition Attitudes In A University Community," *Journal of Nutrition Education*, 7:60-64, August, 1975.

"When To Start Dieting—At Birth," *Medical World News*, 14:31-35, September 7, 1975.

"Will a Fat Baby Become a Fat Child?" *Nutrition Review*, 35:138-140, June, 1977.

Winick, Myron, "Fetal Malnutrition and Growth Processes," *Hospital Practice*, 5:33-41, May, 1970.

Wyse, Bonita, et al., "Nutritional Quality Index Identifies Consumer Nutrient Needs," *Food Technology*, 30:22-40, January, 1976.

Zeigler, H. P., "Oral Satisfaction and Obesity: The Sensual Feel of Food," *Psychology Today*, 9:62-64, 66, August, 1975.

## TEST QUESTIONS

### Multiple Choice Items

1. Shortage of iodine in the diet is an important factor in the: (a) Inability to see in dim light or the symptoms of night blindness, (b) Impaired function of the digestive system, (c) Development of nutritional anemia, (d) *Enlargement of the thyroid gland*, (e) Disruption of the skin.

2. One good source of protein is: (a) Sugar, (b) *Eggs*, (c) Butter, (d) Bread, (e) Vegetables.

3. Which vitamin contributes to the health of the skin and aids in maintaining resistance to infection and is best obtained from butter, vegetables and whole milk: (a) *Vitamin A*, (b) Riboflavin, (c) Ascorbic Acid, (d) Vitamin D, (e) Niacin.

4. The principle use that the body makes of proteins is:

(a) For quick energy, (b) To aid digestion, (c) *For growth and replacement of tissues*, (d) To add bulk to the diet and thus prevent constipation, (e) To stimulate the flow of bile.

5. The most prevalent, as well as the most serious, form of malnutrition in the world today is, (a) Calorie deficiency, (b) Calorie excess, (c) Vitamin deficiency, (d) Mineral deficiency, (e) *Protein deficiency.*

6. If not used by the body immediately, the excess of most vitamins are not stored, but given off in the urine. The exceptions are: (a) *The fat soluble vitamins*, (b) The complex vitamins that are manufactured in the intestine by intestinal flora, (c) The water soluble vitamins, (d) Ascorbic acid, (e) Niacin.

7. Which of the following methods of losing weight is the least dangerous? (a) One week of formula diet such as Metracal, (b) One week of fasting, (c) Two weeks of eating only boiled eggs, (d) *One week of eating one meal a day*, (e) Two weeks of eating only one meal a day.

8. The most common cause of food poisoning in the United States is: (a) Viruses, (b) Botulism, (c) *Staphylococcus*, (d) Amoeba, (e) Protozoa.

9. Protein is supplied least adequately in which of the following foods? (a) Bread, (b) Milk, (c) Nuts, (d) *Fresh fruits*, (e) Cereal.

10. Surplus calories are stored in the body as: (a) Minerals, (b) *Fat*, (c) Proteins, (d) Vitamins, (e) Carbohydrates.

11. The body can store a large amount of Vitamin: (a) *A*, (b) B, (c) C, (d) D, (e) E.

12. Which of the following is *least* true concerning the phenomenon of overweight? (a) The percentage is about the same for both men and women, (b) *The vast majority of overweight cases are caused by glandular malfunction*, (c) Overeating is a primary cause, (d) Obesity is a more advanced form of overweightedness, (e) Exercise plays an important role in the control of body weight.

13. The two nutrients most frequently deficient in American diets are: (a) *Iron and Calcium*, (b) Phosphorus and

Iron, (c) Iodine and Iron, (d) Copper and Calcium, (e) Calcium and Phosphorus.

14. All but which of the following statements are recognized as nutrition myths: (a) Impoverished soils in the United States produce inferior food and subsequent malnutrition, (b) *Foods are the best source of vitamins and minerals*, (c) Most diseases are caused by faulty diets, (d) Overprocessing devitalizes our food and contributes to malnutrition, (e) Most Americans suffer from subclinical deficiencies that are curable by dietary supplementation.

15. What percent over the recommended level for one's specific height, age, and sex is considered overweight: (a) 5 percent, (b) *10 percent*, (c) 15 percent, (d) 20 percent, (e) 25 percent.

16. Nearly a dozen varieties of the B vitamin have been discovered. Which of the following is *not* one of the B complex vitamins? (a) Riboflavin, (b) Niacin, (c) *Ascorbic acid*, (d) Thiamine, (e) Nicotinic acid.

17. The first step in any recommended program to lose or gain weight is to: (a) Conduct a personal caloric intake and expenditure analysis, (b) Purchase an adequate supply of vitamin pills and mineral supplements, (c) *Have a thorough health examination*, (d) Eliminate refined sugars from the diet, (e) Buy a reducing device such as a reducing belt or a machine.

18. All of the following are usually typical of obese people except: (a) *They are more independent and better able to handle stress*, (b) They have little ability to withstand self-deprivation, (c) They are not well accepted by their peers, (d) They are frequently underachievers, (e) They are passive and easy to sway.

19. All of the following can cause colon irritation except: (a) Excessive amounts of coffee, (b) Coarse, fibrous foods, (c) Intestinal infections, (d) Tension, (e) *Excessive amounts of water*.

20. In the United States the only infection that is commonly spread by food is: (a) Typhoid, (b) Dysentery, (c) *Staphylococcus*, (d) Tuberculosis, (e) Diphtheria.

21. All of the following are myths except: (a) All diseases

are due to faulty diets, (b) *Shellfish may be a source of poison during specific seasons of the year*, (c) Processed food is not nutritious, (d) Depleted soils produce depleted foods, (e) Raw foods are best for health.

22. Over a short period of time, the different types of reducing regimens are rarely helpful except: (a) Formula diets, (b) Protein diets, (c) Non-caloric sweeteners, (d) *Salt and water free diet*, (e) Pills and nostrums.

23. All of the following are etiological factors for obesity except: (a) Habit, (b) *Geographic location*, (c) Cultural influences, (d) Psychological factors, (e) Endocrine disorders.

24. Vitamins act as co-enzymes in the body to: (a) Speed up or help with chemical processes of digestion, (b) *Speed up or help with metabolic functions*, (c) Provide energy, (d) Speed up or help with chemical process of blood clotting, (e) Maintain blood pressure.

25. The measurement of energy required for the body to carry on the physiological processes is the: (a) Calorie, (b) Kinetic energy, (c) Nutritional status, (d) *Basal metabolism*, (e) Vital index.

## Matching Items

1. Saturated fats (b)
2. Fat soluble Vitamin C (g)
3. Goiter (e)
4. Amino Acids (a)
5. Found in 1 out of 5 people over 30 (h)
6. Decreases with age (c)
7. Water soluble vitamins (d)
8. Regulate body processes (j)
9. Lack of appetite (f)
10. Disorder of upper intestinal tract (i)

a. Proteins
b. Atherosclerosis
c. Caloric Needs
d. Vitamins C and B Complex
e. Iodine
f. Anorexia
g. Vitamins A, D, E, and K
h. Overweight
i. Gastritis
j. Minerals
k. None of these

## Essay Items

1. What are the varied motivational factors related to food intake?

2. Describe the basic food groups and their contributions to good nutrition.

3. What are some of the typical approaches used by food cultists?

4. How does the Federal Food, Drug, and Cosmetic Act protect the consumer?

5. Why do so many people fail in their dieting and weight loss attempts?

6. What are some current findings and implications on the relationship of nutrition to prenatal development of the fetus?

7. What are some current findings and implications on the relationship of malnutrition and learning disabilities?

8. Discuss some practical guidelines for effective weight control.

9. What diseases can be cured by a proper diet?

# EMOTIONAL HEALTH

*Part Two &ε Chapter 10*

---

## BEHAVIORAL OBJECTIVES

The Student

- identifies the wants, wishes, and desires that effectively guide behavior

- evaluates adequate means of coping with life's situations

- analyzes sources of frustration

- detects conflictual situations

- practices desirable mechanisms for coping with frustrations and conflictual situations

- appraises personal strengths and weaknesses

# SUPPLEMENTARY TEACHING AIDS

## Films

*But Jack Was a Good Driver,* color, 14 min. This film attempts to set the stage for discussion whereby students may share their anxieties and information about suicide. The emphasis is on adolescent suicide and insensitivies of society—family, friends, teachers—to problems affecting adolescents. CRM Educational Films, Del Mar, Calif. 92014.

*On the Move,* color, 27 min. Conflicting life styles and future shock is now. One of four American families moves each year. This film presents family problems associated with moving and alternatives for coping with the stress. Association-Sterling Films, 6644 Sierra Lane, Dublin, Calif. 94566, and 7838 San Fernando Road, Sun Valley, Calif. 91352.

*People Who Care,* color, 25 min. A dramatic film of the life of a young housewife during her mental illness. Withdrawn from her husband and children, she finds there are people who care and want to help. Contemporary Films, McGraw-Hill, 828 Custer Ave., Evanston, Ill. 60202.

*Suicide,* a basic library of 10 books, 12 pamphlets, and reviews of films. $40.00. Mental Health Materials Center, 419 Park Avenue South, New York, N. Y. 10016.

*Time for Growing,* color, 29 min. Understanding growth and development of children requires a good deal of insight, and this unique film takes the viewer into a second-grade classroom situation where the emotional needs and problems of each child can be observed. Metropolitan Life Insurance Company, Health and Welfare Division, One Madison Avenue, New York, N. Y. 10010.

## Filmstrips

*Pre-Retirement Series,* three 10-minute filmstrips. Three filmstrips designed to help those nearing retirement make realistic plans during their working years. The transition into retirement, financial problems often faced by retirees, and what to do with more leisure time are the topics discussed. Association-Sterling Films, 600 Grand Avenue, Ridgefield, N.J. 07657.

**Transparency Originals (See Part 3 of Handbook)**

# ORGANIZATIONS THAT HAVE MATERIALS *

American Guidance Service, Inc., Publisher's Building, Circle Pines, Minnesota 55014 (23 illustrated paperbacks, *The Coping With* series).

American Medical Association, Bureau of Health Education, 535 N. Dearborn St., Chicago, Ill. 60610.

American Schizophrenia Foundation, 56 West 45th St., New York, N. Y. 10036.

Mental Health Foundation Inc. of America, 2 East 86th St., New York, N. Y. 10028.

Mental Health Materials Center, 419 Park Ave., S., New York, N. Y. 10016.

National Association for Mental Health, 1800 N. Kent St., Alexandria, Va. 22209.

National Institutes of Mental Health, 5600 Fishers Lane, Rockville, Md. 20852.

The Hogg Foundation for Mental Health, Publications Division, University of Texas, Austin, Tex. 78712.

*The addresses of these organizations and their policies concerning the sending of materials are subject to change without notice.*

---

# STUDENT INVOLVEMENT

## Investigations

Evaluate personal, weekly activities to determine if more time is needed for socially acceptable methods of reducing tension (hobbies, sports, physical exercise of some type, socializing).

Check how frequently you resort to rationalizing, scapegoating, projecting, compensating, or withdrawing to cope with situations.

Conduct research on the various types of counseling services available in the community on an out-patient basis.

Develop an annotated bibliography on nonprofessional psychological references and periodicals available in the college library.

Make a weekly twenty-four hour schedule of activities that must be accomplished and the amount of time needed to complete these activities.

List some of the extraneous stimuli that personally are annoying (for example, slow drivers, inadequate parking spots, or inconsiderate family and friends) and plan the ways to reduce their frustrating effects with concomitant decrease in tension.

## Action

Initiate a "relaxation class" through the college health and physical education department. See Edmund Jacobson's methods of relaxation, *You Must Relax*, McGraw-Hill, 1962.

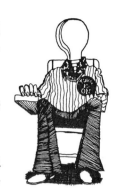

Join a group, if this service is available, for discussions at the college counseling center.

Survey your community's mental health facilities. Are there walk-in clinics, a Suicide Prevention Center, available psychiatrists, psychologists, family or individual counselors? What services are needed, and do they exist in your community?

Volunteer as a tutor for needy children. Help with school work or just be a big brother or big sister that they can talk to.

---

## BASIC SOURCE MATERIALS

Ashby, Neal, "Stop Putting Up with Put-Downs," *Today's Health*, 53:15-19, July-August, 1975.

Brodsky, Carvel, M., "Suicide Attributed to Work," *Suicide and Life-Threatening Behavior*, 7:216-29, Winter, 1977.

Bunnett, Nancy H., "Parental Financial Support and the Financial and Family Problems of College Freshmen," *The Journal of College Student Personnel*, 16:145-148, March, 1975.

Burg, Bob, "The Puzzle of the Psychic Patient," *Human Behavior*, 4:25-30, September, 1975.

Cangemi, Joseph, and Carl Martray, "Awareness: A Psychological Requisite for the Actualizing Personality," *Psychology*, 12:44-49, August, 1975.

Cherlin, Andrew, and Leo Reeder, "The Dimensions of Psychological Well-Being," *Sociological Methods and Research*, 4:189-214, November, 1975.

Clay, Vidal, "Children Deal with Death," *The School Counselor*, 23:175-183, January, 1976.

"Development of Self-Control," *Feelings and Their Medical Significance*, 17:1-4, May-June, 1975.

Feigenberg, Loman, "Care and Understanding of the Dying: A Patient-Centered Approach," *Journal of Death and Dying*, 6:81-94, 1975.

Gould, Roger, "Adult Life Stages—Growth toward Self Tolerance" *Psychology Today*, 8:74-78, February, 1975.

Greenberg, Jerrold S., "Stress, Relaxation, and the Health Educator," *Journal of School Health*, 47:522-25, November, 1977.

Harlow, Harry F., *Learning to Love*, San Francisco: Albion Publishing Company, 1971.

Howard, Jane, *Please Touch*, New York: McGraw-Hill, 1970.

Huang, Ken, "Campus Mental Health: The Foreigner at Your Desk," *Journal of the American College Health Association*, 25:216-219, February, 1977.

Krieger, G. W., and Bascue, L. O., "Terminal Illness: Counseling with a Family Perspective, *The Family Coordinator*," 24:351-55, July, 1975.

Kubler-Ross, Elizabeth, *On Death and Dying*, New York: Macmillan, 1969.

Lair, Jess, *I Ain't Much Baby — But I'm All I've Got*, New York: Doubleday, 1973.

Lamott, Kenneth, *Escape from Stress*, New York: Berkley Publishing Company, 1976.

McGreevy, Abigail, and Judy Van Henkebein, "Crying: The Neglected Dimension," *The Canadian Nurse*, 72:18-20, January, 1976.

Parness, Estelle, "Effects of Experiences with Loss and Death among Preschool Children," *Children Today*, 4:2-7, November-December, 1975.

Savitz, Harry, "Mental Health and Aging," *Mental Hygiene*, 58:21-22, Summer, 1974.

Staples, Robert, "To Be Young, Black and Oppressed," *The Black Scholar*, 7:2-9, December, 1975.

Trotter, Robert J., "Preventing Psychopathology, Preventing Emotional Distress," *Science News*, 108:90-91, August 9, 1975.

Vattano, Anthony J., "Self-Management Procedures for Coping with Stress," *Social Work*, 23:113-19, March, 1978.

*Victiminology — An Instructional Journal*, 2:460-70, 1977-78. Entire issue of 24 articles on family violence and wife beating. Nine book reviews on wife beating.

Zimbardo, Philip, et al., "The Social Disease Called Shyness," *Psychology Today*, 8:69-70, 72, May 1975.

# TEST QUESTIONS

## Multiple Choice Items

1. A workable definition of good mental health includes the concept of being: (a) Like the majority, (b) Independent, (c) Without frustrations, (c) *Adaptable and realistic*, (e) Dependent.

2. A person who attributes his motives to other's behav-

ior is using the adjustive technique of: (a) Rationalization, (b) Suppression, (c) Identification, (d) *Projection,* (e) Repression.

3. One who is mentally healthy: (a) Doesn't deviate in his pattern of behavior, (b) Conforms to the normal or typical, (c) Has few problems, (d) *Has learned to cope effectively with himself and his environment,* (e) Never expresses emotion.

4. With adolescence, status most frequently becomes tied up with the attaining of: (a) Virtue and values, (b) Recognition and skill, (c) Trust and honesty, (d) Initiative and ego, (e) *Independence and self-sufficiency.*

5. Whenever anything occurs to disrupt motivated behavior, the individual is said to be: (a) Maladjusted, (b) Inhibited, (c) *Frustrated,* (d) Autonomous, (e) Assertive.

6. Excusing or justifying failures or shortcomings by explanations that seem to relieve the individual of a responsibility or blame is an example of a defense mechanism called: (a) Suppression, (b) Withdrawal, (c) Substitution, (d) *Rationalization,* (e) Repression.

7. Displaced aggression may result in blaming an innocent person for certain frustrations. This is called: (a) *Scapegoating,* (b) Seclusion, (c) Thwarting, (d) Fantasy, (e) Inhibition.

8. The desire to belong is: (a) The mark of a blind follower of cults and creeds, (b) A symptom of adjustment by retreat, (c) A symptom of adjustment by repression of individuality, (d) *A deep-seated emotional need of all people,* (e) A symptom of mental instability.

9. Which is not an example of a conflict situation: (a) Approach-Approach, (b) Approach-Avoidance, (c) Avoidance-Avoidance, (d) Double Approach-Avoidance, (e) *Approach—Reproach.*

10. Selective forgetting of unpleasant experiences is best described as: (a) Withdrawal, (b) Regression, (c) Substitution, (d) *Repression,* (d) compensation.

11. The development of effective coping behavior has been called: (a) *Adjustment,* (b) Thwarting, (c) Frustration, (d) Conflict, (e) Rationalization.

12. The thwarting of desires or needs brought about by factors that interfere with normal and immediate adjustment of the individual best describes the term: (a) Repression, (b) Stress, (c) Withdrawal, (d) *Frustration*, (e) Maladjustment.

13. Which of the following best describes the affiliate motives? They are: (a) *Socially oriented*, (b) Centered in personal interests, (c) Physiological in nature, (d) Prestige oriented, (e) Competitive in nature.

14. The return to a former, somewhat primitive and rather childish type of behavior, as exemplified by crying when one doesn't get one's way, is a description of the adjustment or defense mechanism of: (a) Repression, (b) Fantasy, (c) Compensation, (d) Displacement, (e) *Regression*.

15. Behaviors of concern to psychological health are: (a) Set early in life and remain unchangeable, (b) Set early in life and of little consequence in coping with life situations, (c) *Learned, and ineffective behavior can be modified by learning*, (d) Learned, and ineffective behavior must be accepted as unchangeable, (e) Unlearned, and ineffective behavior cannot be modified.

16. A classification system that helps to understand motives is: (a) The affiliation-oriented and the social-oriented, (b) *The affiliation-oriented and the prestige-oriented*, (c) The success-oriented and the social-oriented, (d) The personal-oriented and the social-oriented, (e) The affiliation-oriented and the success-oriented.

17. Harlow's studies with young monkeys demonstrated the: (a) *Affectional motives*, (b) Success motives, (c) Task-oriented motives, (d) Prestige-oriented motives, (e) Physical-oriented motives.

18. As a child grows, a conflict frequently develops between: (a) The prestige-oriented and the task-oriented motives, (b) *The prestige-oriented and the affectional relationship*, (c) The affectional motives and the task-oriented motives, (d) The prestige-oriented and esteem motives, (e) The prestige-oriented and status motives.

19. Mechanisms are habit patterns that: (a) *Are routinized*

*through being reinforced and repeated,* (a) Are so strongly entrenched that they cannot be changed, (c) Are so variable in any individual that no pattern can be established, (d) Are developed only in psychoneurotic adjustment, (e) Are an identifying characteristic of certain individuals and not others.

20. The typical reaction to a situation that threatens one's self-esteem or prestige is: (a) Regression, (b) Aggression, (c) Rationalization, (d) Daydreaming, (e) *Withdrawal.*

## Matching Items

1. Interference with motivated behavior (c)
2. Emotional immaturity (e)
3. Reaction to frustration (i)
4. "Sour grapes" (f)
5. Overdevelopment of a behavior (h)
6. Wants, wishes, desires, and purposes (a)
7. Association with another (j)
8. Forgetting of unpleasant experiences (g)
9. Disruption of motivated behavior (b)
10. Behavior in two incompatible ways (d)

a. Motives
b. Frustration
c. Thwarting
d. Conflict
e. Regression
f. Rationalization
g. Repression
h. Compensation
i. Aggression
j. Identification

## Essay Items

1. Briefly describe the essential characteristics of the two groups of social motives—affiliation oriented and prestige oriented.

2. What are some of the status symbols of today's college student? Do they differ from past generations? Are basic needs for status present in all people? In what way do fads and society in general affect status needs and the meeting of those needs? How has Madison Avenue benefited by knowing these basic status needs in people? What effect has it had in meeting the status needs of young people?

3. Frustration can be produced by a variety of situations. What is meant by frustration by delay? By thwarting? By conflict?

4. Explain the term *valence* in relation to response and avoidance.

5. Identify some sound psychological health principles that might be most valuable for college students.

6. How might a college student cope with loneliness and depression? How do moods influence career and life decisions?

# PSYCHOLOGICAL PROBLEMS

*Part Two* e̷ *Chapter* **11**

---

## BEHAVIORAL OBJECTIVES

The Student

- recognizes the extent of mental illness and its associated problems

- can give examples of how psychoneurotic disorders may serve socially useful functions for the individual

- illustrates how physical symptoms may derive from essentially psychological causes

- can give examples of how treatment of minor psychological disorders can be quite successful

- identifies those symptoms which are indications of poor mental adjustment and good mental adjustment

- describes how severe disorders are amenable to treatments of various kinds when therapy is instituted early

# SUPPLEMENTARY TEACHING AIDS

*A Little Slow*, color, 14 min. Ordinary citizen's rights may be denied to people who are mildly retarded. This short film tells the story of two such people, Billy and Carol, who are mildly mentally retarded teenagers. Associated-Sterling Films, 600 Grand Avenue, Ridgefield, N.J. 07657.

*Opening Doors to Mental Health*, color, 30 min. The purpose of this film is to show lay audiences and new staff personnel how a modern mental hospital functions in returning patients to the community. The film follows one patient from admittance and examination through recommended therapy to recovery and eventual return to her family. It shows what can be done in a modern mental health care center, and may be used as a model for community groups who are planning such facilities. Nebraska Psychiatric Institute, Communications Division, 602 S. 44th Ave., Omaha, Neb. 68105.

*Superfluous People*, b / w 60 min. The film discusses welfare aid as a material and moral problem. It pictures various people who need help, and interviews some in order to point out their mental attitudes. Social workers, clergymen, authors, educators and city planners discuss society's neglect of needy citizens. C.B.S. Education and Publishing, 383 Madison Ave., New York, N.Y. 10017.

*To Be Somebody, Again,* color, 19 min. A look at the lives of two individuals who are afflicted by mental illness and at the help given them by their families and by the community mental health center. Sensitively deals with the topic of mental illness in today's stressful world. Association-Sterling Films, 600 Grand Avenue, Ridgefield, N.J. 07657.

*When in Pain*, color, 15 min. Although we avoid pain, it has a physiological and psychological function. Responses to the pain of anxiety, fear, distrust, frustration, and ridicule are explained. A dramatic, very informative film. Malibu Films Inc., P. O. Box 428, Malibu, Calif. 90265.

WRITE FOR SPECIAL CATALOG, National Association for Mental Health, 10 Columbus Circle, New York, N. Y. 10019.

WRITE FOR SPECIAL CATALOG, CRM Educational Films, Del Mar, Calif. 92014. Request descriptions of the following films:

*Aging*
*Frustration / Anger*
*Therapy—What Do You Want Me to Say*
*Depression: A Study in Abnormal Behavior*
*Fifth Street: Skid Row*
*Prejudice: Causes, Consequences, Cures*
*Emotional Development: Aggression*

Transparency Originals (See Part 3 of Handbook)

## ORGANIZATIONS THAT HAVE MATERIALS *

American Psychoanalytic Association, 1 East 57th St., New York, N. Y. 10022.

American Public Health Association, 1015 18th St., N. W., Washington, D. C. 20036.

National Institute of Mental Health, 5600 Fishers Lane, Rockville, Md. 20852.

Schizophrenics Anonymous, American Schizophrenia Foundation, 56 West 45 St., New York, N. Y. 10036.

The Hogg Foundation for Mental Health, Publications Division, The University of Texas, Austin, Tex. 78712.

The President's Committee on Mental Retardation, Washington, D. C. 20201.

*The addresses of these organizations and their policies concerning the sending of materials are subject to change without notice.*

## STUDENT INVOLVEMENT

### Investigations

What significant events have changed the public attitude toward mental illness?

What are the current professional psychological views on "spontaneous recovery" from schizophrenia?

It has been stated that many of the older patients in mental institutions are not really mentally ill, but are placed there because elsewhere they are a burden to their families or society. How true might this be?

How valid is Scientology as treatment for mental illness?

How have drugs changed treatment procedures for mental illness? What opposition is there to sedation of patients and the use of electroshock therapy?

What are the theories and comparisons of an LSD trip and schizophrenia?

## Action

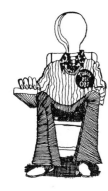

Arrange to tutor a child who has special learning or emotional problems.

Survey community facilities available for various types of treatment: inpatient, out-patient, walk-in clinics, day care, night live-in care, etc.

Male students—volunteer to be a Big Brother through the local Police Boys Club. Help prevent emotional problems with children who have no close, constant male identity role figure (i.e., no father or big brother who cares).

Contact a mental hospital and ask to present periodic music and dance sessions in adolescent and / or children's units.

Volunteer as a recreation leader, musician, companion, or even office worker at a state or private mental hospital. Comment on the problems and quality of care provided by the selected facility.

## BASIC SOURCE MATERIALS

Arehart, Joan, "Mental Patterns of Disease," *Human Behavior*, 5:40-43, January, 1976.

Axline, Virginia L., *Dibs—In Search of Self*, New York: Ballantine Books, 1964.

Beck, Aaron, Maria Kovacs, and Arlene Weissman, "Hopelessness: An Indicator of Suicidal Risk," *Suicide*, 5:98-103, Summer, 1975.

Blackwell, Barbara L., "The Principles of Evaluation," *Community Mental Health Journal*, 13:175-187, Summer 1977.

Casady, Margie, "Character Lasts: If You're Active and Savvy at 30, You'll Be Warm and Witty at 70," *Psychology Today*, 9:138, November, 1975.

Castelli, Jones, "I'm So Lonesome I Could Die," *U.S. Catholic*, 41:32-38, January, 1976.

Delbordge, Patricia, "Identifying the Suicidal Person in the Community," *Nursing Digest*, 3:36-39, November-December, 1975.

Dohnenwend, Bruce, "Sociocultural and Social-Psychological Factors in the Genesis of Mental Disorders," *Journal of Health and Social Behavior*, 16:365-92, December, 1975.

Dyer, Wayne C., *Your Erroneous Zones*, New York: Avon, 1977.

Frankl, Viktor E., *Man's Search for Meaning*, New York: Washington Square Press, 1969.

Gardner, Charles, and Vivian Cadden, "When Someone You Love Is Breaking Down," *McCalls*, 102: 40-48, July, 1975.

Halper, H. P., "Public Acceptance of the Mentally Ill: An Exploration of Attitudes, *Public Health Reports*, 84:59-64, January, 1969.

John, E. Roy, "How the Brain Works— A New Theory," *Psychology Today*, 9:48-52, May, 1976.

Klagsbrun, Francine, "Preventing Teenage Suicide," *Family Health*, 9:21-24, April, 1977.

Lunde, Donald T., "Our Murder Boom," *Psychology Today*, 9:35-42, July, 1975.

McWhirter, Jeffries, "A Parent Education Group in Learning Disabilities," *Journal of Learning Disabilities*, 9:16-20, January, 1976.

Marsh, Stephen, Melinda Peters, Tom Peters, and Ralph Stewart, "An Object-Relations Approach to Psychotherapy with Marital Couples, Families, and Children," *Family Process*, 14:161-178, June, 1975.

McNeely, James D., Mohammad Shafii, and John J. Schwab. "The Student Suicide Epidemic,"

*Today's Education*, 66:70-73, September-October 1977.

Myers, Jerome K., et al., "Life Events, Social Integration and Psychiatric Symptomatology," *Journal of Health and Social Behavior*, 16:421-27, December, 1975.

Nathanson, James, and Paul Greengard "Second Messengers in the Brain," *Scientific American*, 237:108-119, August, 1977.

Ries, Janet K., "Public Acceptance of the Disease Concept of Alcoholism," *Journal of Health and Social Behavior*, 18:338-344, September, 1977.

Shapiro, Rodney, "Problems in Teaching Family Therapy," *Professional Psychology*, 6:41-44, February, 1975.

Siegler, Miriam, and Humphry Osmond, "Models of Madness: Mental Illness Is Not Romantic," *Psychology Today*, 8:71-72, 75-76, 78, November, 1974.

Tolar, Calvin J., "The Mental Health of Students: Do Teachers Hurt or Help?" *Journal of School Health*, 45:71-75, February, 1975.

"The Unwanted Child," *Science News*, 108:168, September 13, 1975.

Wallerstein, J.,et al., "The Effects of Parental Divorce: Experiences of the Preschool Child," *Journal of the American Academy of Child Psychiatry*, 14:600-16, Autumn, 1975.

Whittington, H. G., and Charles Steinbarger, "Preliminary Evaluation of a Decentralized Community Mental Health Clinic," *American Journal of Public Health*, 60:64-77, January, 1970.

## TEST QUESTIONS
### Multiple Choice Items

1. Approximately how many million Americans are mentally or emotionally disturbed and in need of psychiatric treatment? (a) 10 million, (b) *20 million*, (c) 30 million, (d) 40 million, (e) 50 million.

2. Anxiety reaction, a form of neurosis, is characterized by: (a) *Constant feeling of impending disaster*, (b) Constant feeling of being persecuted, (c) Numerous phobias, (d) A desire to be alone, (e) Loss of consciousness.

3. The most common major mental disorder is: (a) *Schizophrenia*, (b) Manic depression, (c) Paranoia, (d) Neurasthenia, (e) Psychasthenia.

4. The psychosis of general paresis is a direct result of the disease: (a) Tuberculosis, (b) Cerebral hemorrhage, (c) *Syphilis*, (d) Alcoholism, (e) Smallpox.

5. Neurasthenia literally means: (a) Hysteria, (b) *A nervous weakness*, (c) Fatigue, (d) Anxiety, (e) Psychotic behavior.

6. The relationship between the mind and the body is called: (a) Psychological, (b) Psychiatric, (c) Physiological, (d) *Psychosomatic*, (e) Neurotic.

7. All of the following are forms of dissociative reactions except: (a) Amnesias, (b) Fugues, (c) Dual or multiple personalities, (d) *Belligerence*, (e) Somnambulism.

8. Psychoanalysis is best defined as: (a) A means of interpreting behavior in terms of repressed sexual conflicts, (b) *A procedure of bringing unconscious conflicts into consciousness*, (c) a means whereby present conflicts may be resolved in terms of organic disturbance, (d) An analysis by a medical expert of the interrelationship between biological and social egos, (e) A way of interpreting the relationship between the mind and the body.

9. A classical symptom or form of psychasthenia is: (a) hallucinations, (b) Delusions, (c) Amnesias, (d) Melancholia, (e) *Phobias*.

10. Freud introduced a theory some years ago by announcing that neuroses were caused by: (a) Extreme introversion, (b) Lack of social adjustment, (c) *Sexual frustration*, (d) Use of adjustment mechanisms, (e) Failure to use mechanisms.

11. All of these conditions are most commonly recognized as psychosomatic in nature except: (a) Common al-

lergies, (b) Ulcers, (c) Colitis, (d) Hypertension, (e) *Viral infections.*

12. Neuroses are best characterized by: (a) *The inability to react normally to certain life situations,* (b) Gradual mental deterioration, (c) Antisocial tendencies, (d) Suicidal tendencies, (e) Severe mental retardation.

13. Which would be the least likely way to treat a neurosis: (a) Medical, (b) Psychological, (c) Sociological, (d) Chemotherapeutic, (e) *Institutionalizing.*

14. Motor, sensory, and epileptic symptoms may be produced by the mental illness: (a) Phobia, (b) Asthenia, (c) Obsession, (d) *Hysteria,* (e) Paranoia.

15. Historically, four subgroups of schizophrenia have been recognized. Which does *not* fit into this category: (a) Simple, (b) *Manic,* (c) Paranoid, (d) Hebephrenic, (e) Catatonic.

16. A phobia is a neurosis best characterized by: (a) Repetitive actions, (b) Physical ailments, (c) Persistent thoughts, (d) Suicidal tendencies, (e) *Morbid fears.*

17. Psychoses usually can be produced by all but: (a) Infectious diseases, (b) Brain tumors, (c) *High blood pressure,* (d) Nutritional deficiencies, (e) Meningitis.

18. Antisocial personalities are characterized by: (a) Neurotic traits, (b) *A marked deficiency in ethical and moral development,* (c) Hallucinations, (d) A marked change in personality, (e) Highly intelligent individuals.

19. Which is *least* likely to be considered a form of adjustment by ailment: (a) Malingering, (b) Headaches, (c) Upset stomach, (d) Desire for attention, (e) *Desire for more responsibility.*

20. Emotionally sick individuals that suffer from unreasonable fears, obsessions, depressed feelings, and compulsions are usually referred to as: (a) Psychotic, (b) Vagrants, (c) Insane, (d) *Psychoneurotic,* (e) Manic-depressives.

## Matching Items

1. Persistent thoughts (c)
2. Pathological fears (e)
3. Psychoneurotic behavior (h)
4. Sleepwalking (b)
5. Disorders of perception (f)
6. Inability to recall (a)
7. Nervous disorder (j)
8. Disease of the mind (i)
9. Repetitive actions (d)
10. False beliefs (g)

a. Amnesia
b. Somnambulism
c. Obsessions
d. Compulsions
e. Phobias
f. Hallucinations
g. Delusions
h. Hysteria
i. Psychosis
j. Neurosis

## Essay Items

1. Show how psychosomatic disorders exemplify the unity of the physical and the mental. Give examples.

2. Schizophrenia and manic-depression are both examples of a psychosis. Describe the differences between them. Consider their prognosis, nature, and possible causes.

3. Why do phobias often require medical assistance?

4. Describe the difference between a neurosis and a psychosis.

5. How has society changed in consideration of individuals with mental problems?

6. Children are able to adjust to many trying and traumatic situations. However, there are some conditions where "normal adjustment" may be prohibitive. What are some mental illnesses that affect children, and what are their possible causes?

7. How might communities provide medical care to people who are seriously ill with a mental disease, but not in need of institutional care or for whom this type of care might be more harmful than beneficial?

# ALCOHOL AND TOBACCO

*Part Two* ℰ *Chapter 12*

---

## BEHAVIORAL OBJECTIVES

The Student

- identifies the physical and social values of the appropriate use of alcohol as a beverage

- illustrates how the drinking of alcoholic beverages is an accepted cultural practice in the United States

- analyzes the emotionalism arising out of the controversies about if, when, how, where, and by whom, alcoholic beverages should be used

- distinguishes between acceptable and unacceptable drinking patterns

- accepts responsiblity for drinking behavior if the decision is made to use alcohol

- evaluates the serious social problems resulting from the inappropriate use of alcohol

- identifies the relationships between smoking and acute and chronic illness

- draws conclusions from scientific studies about the physiological and psychological effects of smoking

- abstains from smoking

# SUPPLEMENTARY TEACHING AIDS

*A Breath of Air*, color, 20 min. The film presents the relationship of smoking to emphysema and chronic bronchitis. American Lung Association, 1740 Broadway, New York, N.Y. 10019.

*Alcoholism: A Model of Drug Dependency*, color, 20 min., rental. The dependency model is used to explain the behavior of the alcoholic. The isolation and dependency syndrome is explained in developmental terms from childhood to adulthood. Alternate dependency patterns are presented to help the alcoholic break the dependency cycle. CRM Educational Films, Del Mar, Calif. 92014.

*As We See It*, color, 25 min. Some youngsters determined to change their parent's smoking habits produce their own TV documentary, including interviews with physicians and researchers. These smart kids look like professionals in this production and put their message across. American Lung Association, 1740 Broadway, New York, N. Y. 10019.

*The Disease Called Alcoholism*, 15 min. Jellenick's theory and "X" factor theory on causative factors of alcoholism. Pfizer Medical Teaching Film Library, 267 W. 25th St., New York, N. Y. 10016.

*Ins-and-Outs of Alcoholism*. This kit includes a record, reprints, pamphlets. Sandoz Pharmaceuticals, Hanover, N. J. 07936.

*Point of View*, black and white, 19 min. An offbeat, satirical comment on habit of smoking. Discussion guide available. American Lung Association, 1740 Broadway, New York, N. Y. 10019.

Transparency Originals (See Part 3 of Handbook)

## ORGANIZATIONS THAT HAVE MATERIALS *

Al-Anon (for family of alcoholic) (consult telephone directory for local chapter)

Al-Ateen (for teenaged children of alcoholic parents) (consult telephone directory for local chapter)

Alcoholics Anonymous, General Services, P.O. Box 459 Grand Central Station, New York, N. Y. 10017.

American Hospital Association, 840 North Lake Shore Drive, Chicago, Ill. 60611.

American Psychiatric Association, 1700 18th Street, N. W., Washington, D. C. 20009.

Kemper Insurance, Advertising and Public Relations Department, 100 Tenth Ave., Fulton, Ill. 61252.

**National Association of Blue Shield Plans, 840 North Lake Shore Drive, Chicago, Ill. 60611.**

National Clearinghouse for Drug Abuse Information, P.O. Box 1635, Rockville, Md. 20850.

National Council on Alcoholism, 733 Third Ave., New York, N. Y. 10017.

National Womens Christian Temperance Union, 1730 Chicago Ave., Evanston, Ill. 60200.

Rutgers Center of Alcohol Studies, Box 554 Smithers Hall, State University Rutgers, New Brunswick, N. J. 08903.

**Veterans Administration Central Office, 810 Vermont Avenue, N.W., Washington, D. C. 20005.**

*The addresses of these organizations and their policies concerning the sending of materials are subject to change without notice.*

## STUDENT INVOLVEMENT

### Investigations

What is the public community's public school program (in operation) for education in alcohol and tobacco use?

Collect old physiology and hygiene texts. Explain philosophies and approaches used with reference to tobacco and alcohol education.

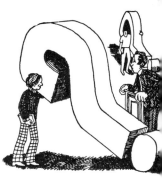

What rehabilitation programs are available in both government and private agencies to work with alcoholics and their families in your home community?

Describe the programs in the community to help the heavy smoker "break the habit."

What does research indicate are the effects of alcohol on the fetus?

What does research indicate are the effects of smoking on the fetus? Does tobacco cause birth defects?

What were the social forces leading to the Prohibition Era, and why was prohibition of alcohol not workable?

Smoking is prohibited in certain occupations. Why? What are some of them?

Contrast the rates of alcoholism between the U.S. and other countries.

## Action

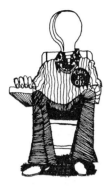

Survey the campus to find the percentage of students who have quit smoking. What were some motivating factors and problems encountered?

Contact the local chapter of the American Cancer Society or American Lung Association for assistance in sponsoring a "Quit Smoking Clinic" on your campus. Advertise well. Good Luck.

Make arrangements with the Student Union to display a wheelbarrow full of cigarette butts. Decorate it with tombstones, posters, etc. for an antismoking campaign. Hand out pamphlets, "Me Quit Smoking? How?" and "Me Quit Smoking? Why?" Available from The American Lung Association, 1790 Broadway, New York, N. Y. 10019.

Stop smoking yourself, if you can.

Survey various groups of people, adults, children, students on their attitude toward alcoholism and the individual alcoholic. What factors might contribute to their attitudes?

Attend several Alcoholics Anonymous meetings. Report your reactions to the class.

Tape record some tobacco and alcohol advertisements. What "psychology" is used to sell the product? Play these in class and survey class response and susceptibility.

## BASIC SOURCE MATERIALS

### Alcohol

"Alcohol and Marijuana—Menace Among Teen-Agers," *U.S. News and World Report*, 79:28-30, November, 1975.

Berland, Theodore, "Should Children Be Taught to Drink?" *Today's Health*, 47:46-50, 83-88, February, 1969.

Fisher, Arthur, "Sober—Yet Drinking Too Much," *New York Times Magazine*, Sec. 6, pp. 16, 65, 72, 76, May 18, 1975.

Goldstein, Michael S., "Drinking and Alcoholism as Presented in College Health Textbooks," *Journal of Drug Education*, 5:109-125, August, 1975.

Horoshak, Irene R.N., "Teen-Age Drinking: A Growing Problem or a Problem of Growing?" *R.N.* 39:63-69, March, 1976.

Johnson, Gordon, "LSD in the Treatment of Alcoholism," *American Journal of Psychiatry*, 126:63-69, October, 1969.

Keller, Mark, "Problems of Epidemiology in Alcohol Problems," *Studies on Alcohol*, 36:1442-1451, November, 1975.

Mann, Marty, *Marty Mann's New Primer on Alcoholism*, New York: Holt, Rinehart and Winston, 1973 (14th printing)

Mikuriya, T. H., "Cannabis Substitution: An Adjunctive Therapeutic Tool in the Treatment of Alcoholism," *Medical Times*, 98:187-191, April, 1970.

Patterson, R. D., "Preventing Self-Destructive Behavior," *Geriatrics*, 29:115-18, 121, 1974.

Shapiro, R. D., "Alcohol, Tobacco, and Illicit Drug Use Among Adolescents," *International Journal Addiction*, 10:387-390, 1975.

Steiner, Claude, *Games Alcoholics Play: The Analysis of Life Scripts*, New York: Grove Press, Inc., 1971.

Veith, Ilza, "Touch Not, Taste Not, Handle Not," *Modern Medicine*, 38:176-182, May 4, 1970.

## Tobacco

"Can Other People's Smoke Hurt You?" *Changing Times*, 29:11-12, September, 1975.

Colley, J., "Passive Smoking in Children," *Nursing Times*, 71:1858-59, 20, November, 1975.

Doyle, Nancy C., "The Facts about Second-Hand Cigarette Smoke," *American Lung Association Bulletin*, 60:13-15, July, 1974.

Godber, George E., "Smoking Disease: A Self-Inflicted Injury," *American Journal of Public Health*, 60:235-242, February, 1970.

Horn, Daniel, "Why People Smoke," *World Health*, 26-31, December, 1975.

Jones, P., "Smoking and Pregnancy," *Nursing Times*, 71:2038-9, December 18, 1975.

Lauder, John, "Third World Conference on Smoking and Health," *Cancer News*, 29:10-15, Fall, 1975.

Mauer, H., and J. Schwartz, "Do Smokers Clinics Really Work?" *Science Digest*, 78:72-6, September, 1975.

Meredith, H. V., "Relationships between Tobacco Smoking of Pregnant Women and Body Size of Offspring," *Human Biology*, 47:451-72, December, 1975.

"No Smoking—Some States Mean It," *U.S. News and World Report*, 79:45, October 20, 1975.

Ottens, Allen J., "The Effort of Transcendental Meditation upon Modifying the Cigarette Smoking Habit," *Journal of School Health*, XLV:577-583, December, 1975.

Pederson, L. L. et al., "Comparison of Hypnosis Plus Counseling, Counseling Alone, and Hypnosis Alone in a Community Service Smoking Withdrawal Program," *Journal of Consulting Clinical Psychology*, 43:920, December, 1975.

"Social Smoking," *Science Digest*, 79:24, January, 1976.

Steinfeld, Jesse L., "There's Even Stronger Evidence on the Health Hazards of Smoking," *American Lung Association Bulletin*, 61:7-4, October, 1975.

Sterling, Theodore D., "A Critical Reassessment of the Evidence Bearing on Smoking as the Cause of Lung Cancer," *American Journal of Public Health*, 65:939-950, September, 1975.

*The Dangers of Smoking, The Benefits of Quitting*, New York: The American Cancer Society, 1972.

Weiss, W., "Smoking and Cancer: A Rebuttal," *American Journal of Public Health*, 65:954-955, September, 1975.

Doyle, Nancy C., "The Facts about Second-Hand Cigarette Smoke," *American Lung Association Bulletin*, 60:13-15, July, 1974.

*The Dangers of Smoking, The Benefits of Quitting*, New York: The American Cancer Society, 1972.

Godber, George E., "Smoking Disease: A Self-Inflicted Injury," *American Journal of Public Health*, 60: 235-242, February, 1970.

Horn, Daniel, "Why People Smoke," *World Health*, 26-31, December, 1975.

Jones, P., "Smoking and Pregnancy," *Nursing Times*, 71:2038-9, December 18, 1975.

Lauder, John, "Third World Conference on Smoking and Health," *Cancer News*, 29:10-15, Fall, 1975.

Mauer, H., and J. Schwartz, "Do Smokers Clinics Really Work?" *Science Digest*, 78:72-6, September, 1975.

Meredith, H. V., "Relationships between Tobacco Smoking of Pregnant Women and Body Size of Offspring," *Human Biology*, 47:451-72, December, 1975.

"No Smoking—Some States Mean It," *U.S. News and World Report*, 79: 45, October 20, 1975.

Ottens, Allen J., "The Effect of Transcendental Meditation Upon Modifying the Cigarette Smoking Habit," *Journal of School Health*, XLV:577-583, December, 1975.

L. L. Pederson, et al., "Comparison of Hypnosis Plus Counseling, Counseling Alone, and Hypnosis Alone in a Community Service Smoking Withdrawal Program," *Journal of Consulting Clinical Psychology*, 43:920, December, 1975.

"Social Smoking," *Science Digest*, 79:24, January, 1976.

Steinfeld, Jesse L., "There's Even Stronger Evidence on the Health Hazards of Smoking," *American Lung Association Bulletin*, 61:7-14, October, 1975.

Sterling, Theodore D., "A Critical Reassessment of the Evidence Bearing on Smoking as the Cause of Lung Cancer," *American Journal of Public Health*, 65:939-950, September, 1975.

"Want to Quit Smoking? Here Are Tested Ways," *Today's Health*, 47:84-86, May, 1969.

Weiss, W., "Smoking and Cancer: A Rebuttal," *American Journal of Public Health*, 65:954-955, September, 1975.

Special materials on smoking education are available from Bureau of Health Education, Center for Disease Control, Atlanta, Georgia, 30333. The national smoking education program has been evaluated and new approaches and materials prepared for schools. For more information write to the Bureau of Health Education.

## Tobacco and Health Hazards

American Cancer Society—contact local chapters.

American College of Chest Physicians,

112 East Chestnut St., Chicago, Illinois 60611.

American Dental Association, Bureau

of Dental Health Education, 211 East Chicago Ave., Chicago, Ill. 60611 (material on smoking and oral cancer).

American Heart Association—contact local chapters.

American Lung Association—contact local chapters.

American Medical Association, 535 Dearborn St., Chicago, Ill. 60610.

National Academy of Pediatrics, 1801 Hinman Ave., Evanston, Ill. 60204.

National Education Association, 1201 16th St., N.W. Washington, D.C. 20036.

National Interagency Council on Smoking and Health, 419 Park Ave., S., New York, N.Y. 10016.

Public Affairs Pamphlets, 381 Park Ave., S., New York, N.Y. 10016.

Smoking and Health Project, American Public Health Association, 1015 18th St., N. W., Washington, D. C. 20036.

U.S. Department of Health, Education and Welfare, National Clearinghouse for Smoking and Health, Center for Disease Control, Atlanta, Ga. 30333.

## TEST QUESTIONS

## Multiple Choice Items

1. An alcoholic "black out" is best described as: (a) Passing out, (b) Temporary blindness, (c) Temporary unconsciousness, (d) *Temporary amnesia*, (e) The inability to learn.

2. "Loss of control" in the alcoholic refers to the loss of the ability to: (a) Control his actions after drinking, (b) Refuse the first drink, (c) *Stop drinking once he starts*, (d) Control whether he takes the first drink, (e) Drink sociably.

3. There are many misconceptions about the use and abuse of alcohol. All of the following are *false* except: (a) An alcoholic is continuously drunk, (b) The alcoholic drinks because he likes the taste, (c) *Some alcoholics drink only beer*, (d) Moderate drinking shortens the life span, (e) Alcohol increases perceptual ability.

4. A true alcoholic can remain well only if he: (a) Learns to drink in moderation, (b) Never drinks alone,

(c) Drinks beer only, (d) *Never drinks,* (e) Receives psychiatric treatment.

5. A symptom of early-stage alcoholism is: (a) Chronic hangover, (b) Gulping and sneaking drinks, (c) Blackouts, (d) Gross drinking behavior, (e) *Loss of control.*

6. The majority of persons probably start using alcoholic drinks because of: (a) Despondency, (b) Excitement, (c) *Social custom,* (d) Craving for a particular beverage, (e) Early use of soft drinks.

7. Alcoholism is now regarded by the experts who study the problem as: (a) A character disorder, (b) A crime, (c) An escape mechanism, (d) *A Physical and / or mental illness,* (e) A moral weakness.

8. Excessive, continued consumption of alcohol usually causes: (a) Kidney infections, (b) *Cirrhosis of the liver,* (c) Cirrhosis of the kidney, (d) Circulatory diseases, (e) Cirrhosis of the stomach.

9. Alcohol consumed by a person accustomed to drinking: (a) Is absorbed more slowly, (b) *Is oxidized more quickly,* (c) Is oxidized more slowly, (d) Is less apt to be toxic, (e) Has no different effects than in a nondrinker.

10. Most people who drink at all, drink because under the influence of alcohol they feel that: (a) They lose some of their inhibitions, (b) They can be more personable, (c) They can relax, (d) They are more socially accepted, (e) *All of these.*

11. The three most widely used methods of rehabilitating the alcoholic are: (a) Isolation, drugs and psychotherapy, (b) *Institutional methods, psychotherapy and drug therapy,* (c) Organizational methods, psychotherapy and isolation, (d) Food deprivation, psychotherapy and organizational methods, (e) Food supplements, detoxification and drug therapy.

12. Which of the following statements is *not* true regarding alcoholics: (a) Alcoholics may possibly have physiological characteristics which predispose them toward alcoholism, (b) Alcoholics are suffering from a disease, (c) The alcoholic has a preoccupation with al-

cohol, (d) The alcoholic rationalizes his drinking behavior, (e) *After a few years of rehabilitation the alcoholic may return to normal social drinking.*

13. The difference between a "heavy drinker" and an alcoholic is: (a) None, (b) The alcoholic has a preoccupation with alcohol, the heavy drinker does not, (c) The alcoholic has the "x" factor, the problem drinker does not, (d) The heavy drinker does not develop a tolerance or ability to "hold his liquor," (e) *The alcoholic has a compulsive desire to drink, the heavy drinker is not compulsive.*

14. Studies on the relationship between smoking and lung cancer by the American Cancer Society show: (a) The same relationship for cigarette smokers, cigar smokers and pipe smokers, (b) A significantly higher death rate for cigar smokers, (c) *A significantly higher rate for heavy cigarette smokers,* (d) No significant relationship, (e) A relationship for men, but not for women.

15. The tiny air sacs in the respiratory system that serve in the exchange of oxygen and carbon dioxide are called the: (a) Bronchioles, (b) Pleura, (c) Epiglotti, (d) *Alveoli,* (e) Mucosi.

16. Breathlessness or a marked shortness of breath is a common symptom of smoking related to the diseases: (a) *Emphysema and chronic bronchitis,* (b) Emphysema and peptic ulcers, (c) Pleurisy and pneumonia, (d) Peptic ulcers and chronic bronchitis, (e) Asthma and allergies.

17. The effect of cigarette smoke, or more specifically nicotine, upon the body is to: (a) *Stimulate and then depress the nervous system,* (b) Lower the blood pressure, (c) Dilate the arteries, (d) Decrease the pulse rate, (e) Raise the temperature of the extremities.

18. Which of the following statements is *least* true regarding smoking: (a) The death rate for excessive users of tobacco is higher than that for non-smokers, (b) *Stopping cigarette smoking after a long exposure is not beneficial,* (c) The non-smoker has a lower incidence of lung cancer than the smoker, (d) Some individuals are tobacco-sensitive, (e) Premature births are greater for smoking mothers than for non-smoking mothers.

19. Cigarette smoke has a direct effect upon the cilia and

mucus of the bronchial tubes which are a part of the respiratory tract's cleansing system. With respect to these structures or processes, which one of the following statements is most accurate: Cigarette smoke: (a) *Paralyzes the cilia action for a period of time*, (b) Produces a marked underproduction of mucus, (c) Shrinks the bronchioles, (d) Increases the action of the cilia, (e) Has no determined effect on the cilia, mucus production, or bronchioles.

20. The statistical evidence that links cigarette smoking to lung cancer: (a) Is inconclusive and unconvincing, (b) *Is strongly suggestive of a causal relationship between the two*, (c) Is insufficient to warrant serious concern on the part of smokers, (d) Is based on unreliable data, (e) Gives a false picture of the situation because it fails to take into account the part played by air pollution in producing lung cancer.

21. Smoking produces certain distinct immediate physiological changes in the body. Which of the following is *least* true regarding these effects: (a) The heart rate increases, (b) Blood flow in the peripheral vessels decreases, (c) The blood sugar level is raised, (d) Blood pressure is elevated, (e) *Pulse rate decreases*.

22. The most probable effect of carbon monoxide on the body, as a product found in cigarette smoke, is that of interfering with normal: (a) Blood oxygenation, (b) Food absorption, (c) Kidney excretion, (d) Sensory perception, (e) Locomotion.

23. A carcinogen is a substance: (a) Used to help prevent mildew on tobacco plants, (b) Added to tobacco as a moisturizing agent, (c) Used as an insecticide, (d) *Related to the cause of cancer*, (e) Classified as a virulent poison.

24. The function of the cilia that line the trachea and bronchial tubes of the respiratory tract is basically to: (a) Effect the gas exchanges, (b) Collect the incoming air from the nose and mouth, (c) Create the voice sounds, (d) *Serve as a filtering system*, (e) Eliminate carbon dioxide.

25. Cigarettes cause chronic cough in most smokers by: (a) *Damaging the cilia*, (b) Damaging the alveoli,

(c) Causing lung cancer, (d) Stimulating the cough center, (e) Depressing the brain.

## Essay Items

1.  Recovery from acute alcoholism is a long and difficult road. Identify five measures utilized to help rehabilitate the alcoholic.

2.  Several million people are classified as alcoholics in the United States. Most of them did not suddenly become so, but passed through various drinking phases. Indicate five of the signs or symptoms that indicate that the person has a drinking problem or is progressing through the stages of alcoholism.

3.  There are many misconceptions and misunderstandings concerning the nature, characteristics, and effects of alcohol. For example, some people still believe that a drink will cure a cold. Indicate five other false beliefs about alcohol and the disease of alcoholism.

4.  Research has revealed the effects of beverage alcohol on the individual. Indicate the physiological effects of heavy or continued drinking on the body. Include reference to some of the more important associated diseases which appear to be more frequent among excessive drinkers of alcohol.

5.  List some of the arguments for and against social drinking. What elements of society support or reject social drinking? If alcohol plays a part in socializing people are there alternate ways of achieving the same desired effects?

6.  What are some of the reasons that cause people to start smoking and why do they continue to smoke?

7.  Briefly describe some of the recent research findings on the relationship between cigarette smoking and coronary heart disease and diseases of the peripheral blood vessels.

8.  Describe some of the findings of research that indicate a relationship between longevity and the smoking of cigarettes.

9. Describe some motivational factors that must be present in order for a person to be successful in his attempts to stop smoking.

# DRUG ABUSE

*Part Two* ✣ *Chapter* 13

---

## BEHAVIORAL OBJECTIVES

**The Student**

- relates basic factual information concerning the nature and characteristics of stimulant, depressant, and hallucinogenic substances

- identifies some of the personal problems related to the abuse of dangerous substances

- critically evaluates misconceptions, beliefs, and information on drugs in order to establish a sound basis for personal action

- indicates certain of the physiological, psychological, economic, social, and cultural problems created by the use of stimulants, hallucinogens, and depressants in modern society

- summarizes some of the efforts being made to scientifically investigate and cope with problems related to the use of various drugs

# SUPPLEMENTARY TEACHING AIDS

*Drug Abuse: Everybody's Hang-Up*, color, 14 min. Designed to heighten awareness of a concern for the problem, this film does not attempt to provide answers, but offers suggestions to adults. Appropriate for lead-in discussion, or as a summarizing film. N.E.A. Sound Studios, 1201 16th St., N.W., Washington, D.C. 20036.

*Trigger Films on Health.* Topics: Alcohol, Drugs. Special 1-3-minute films to stimulate discussion. The audience provides the ending of the film as the film stops suddenly before an episode is completed. University of Michigan Television Center, 400 S. Fourth St., Ann Arbor, Michigan 48103.

Variety of pamphlets and leaflets. Record, "First Vibration," plus anti-drug songs by popular folk singers. Do It Now Foundation, 5115 Phoenix, Arizona 85010.

Transparency Originals (See Part 3 of Handbook)

## ORGANIZATIONS THAT HAVE MATERIALS *

Abbott Laboratories, 14th and Sheridan Road, North Chicago, Ill. 60064.

American Medical Association, Bureau of Health Education, 535 N. Dearborn St., Chicago, Ill. 60610.

American Pharmaceutical Association, 2215 Constitution Ave., N.W., Washington, D.C. 20037.

Charles Pfizer and Company, Inc., 235 E. 42nd St., New York, N.Y. 10017.

Ciba Pharmaceutical Products, Inc., Summit, N.J. 07901.

Do It Now Foundation, P.O. Box 5115, Phoenix, Arizona 85010.

Eli Lilly and Company, Educational Division, 740 S. Alabama St., Indianapolis, Ind. 46205.

E. R. Squibb and Sons, 745 Fifth Ave., New York, N.Y. 10022.

Food and Drug Administration, Dept. Health, Education and Welfare, Washington, D.C. 20025.

Grafton Publications, Inc., 331 Madison Ave., New York, N.Y. 10017, *Addiction and Drug Abuse Report*, monthly newsletter.

Merck, Sharp and Dohme, Public Relations Department, Westpond, Penn. 19486.

Narcotics Education, Inc., 6830 Laurel St., N. W., Washington, D. C. 20012.

National Clearinghouse for Drug Abuse Information, P.O. Box 1635, Rockville, Md. 20850.

National Coordinating Council on Drug Abuse Information, Box 19400, Washington, D.C. 20036, $1.00 for comprehensive listing of materials.

National Institute for Mental Health, 5454 Wisconsin Ave., Chevy Chase, Md. 20203.

National Organization for the Reform of Marijuana Laws, 275 Madison Ave., Suite 1033, New York, N.Y. 10016.

Parke, Davis and Company, P.O. Box 118, E.P. Annex, Detroit, Mich. 48232.

Pharmaceutical Manufacturers Association, Public Relations Division, 1155 15th St., N. W., Washington, D. C. 20005.

Ross Laboratories, 625 Cleveland Ave., Columbus, Ohio 43215.

Smith, Kline, and French Laboratories, 1500 Spring Garden Rd., Philadelphia, Pa. 19130.

The Upjohn Company, Trade Relations Department, 7000 Portage Road, Kalamazoo, Mich. 49002.

*The addresses of these organizations and their policies concerning the sending of materials are subject to change without notice.

## STUDENT INVOLVEMENT

### Investigations

Discuss the "pros and cons" regarding the legalization of marijuana. How has the movement to legalize marijuana progressed in the last ten years?

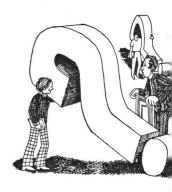

Survey classmates by questionnaire to find out what factual information they know about drug action and drug reactions.

Try to find out the extent of the abuse of narcotics and dangerous drugs in the community, particularly by elementary and junior high school students.

What facilities are available in the community for the treatment of addiction? What facilities might be needed? Make a proposal for facilities to meet the needs. How have budget cuts affected drug treatment programs?

### Action

What medical training do the local emergency squads and / or police have for handling drug emergencies such as barbiturate overdose, amphetamine psychosis, etc.?

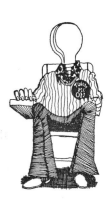

What service exists in your community for poison control? Is there a Poison Control Center? Survey local hospitals to learn how poison cases are handled.

Set up a student-led and operated "Drug Hot Line." Operate in conjunction with other community groups that have drug programs. Offer a "listening ear" advice and referral. (Approach local health department to pay phone bills.) Obtain the services of a physician to sponsor your group and to be available to handle any emergencies.

Display drug information materials and set up a question booth in the student union.

Visit a rehabilitation center for addicts. If possible, interview patients.

Contact the local Board of Education or Physical Education and Health Supervisor. Offer to assist in Drug Abuse Education programs in local high schools.

## BASIC SOURCE MATERIALS

"Abuse of Medicines: Self Medication," *Drug Intelligence and Clinical Pharmacy*, 10:16-33, January, 1976.

Alpert, Richard, Sidney Cohen and Lawrence Schiller, *LSD*, New York: The New American Library, 1966.

"Amphetamine," *Drug Enforcement*, 2:26-29, Winter, 1975.

Ballou, Mary, "Crisis Intervention: A Call for Involvement for the Health Professional," *Journal of School Health*, 47:603-06, December, 1977.

Batalden, Paul, Scott Nelson, and Bowak Wolff, "Manpower Training as an Alternative to Disadvantaged Adolescent Drug Misuse," *American Journal of Public Health*, 65:599-604, June, 1975.

Bloomquist, E. R., *Marijuana*, Toronto: Glencoe Press, 1968.

Boe, Sue, "Drugs: The Tools of Medical Progress," *American Journal of Public Health*, 40:65-70, February, 1970.

Brenner, Berthold, "Enjoyment as A Preventive of Depressive Affect," *Journal of Community Psychology*, 3:346-357, October, 1975.

Byrd, Oliver E., *Medical Readings On Drug Abuse*, Reading, Mass.: Addison-Wesley, 1970.

Carroll, Jerome, "Mental Illness and 'Disease': Outmoded Concepts in Alcohol and Drug Rehabilitation," *Community Mental Health Journal*, 11:418-429, Winter, 1975.

Chambers, Carl D., Walter R. Cuskey, and Arthur D. Moffett, "Demographic Factors in Opiate Addiction Among Mexican-Americans," *Public Health Reports*, 85:523-532, June, 1970.

Cohen, Mark and Joseph Kern, Ronald Sauerlse, and Susan Zitter, "Community Drug Abuse Agencies, An Effective Approach to the Drug Abuse Problem?"*Journal of Community Psychology*, 4:74-80, January, 1976.

D'Andrea, Vincent J., *"Psychoactive Drugs,* Menlo•Park, Calif.: Cummings Publishing Company, 1977.

Dohner, V. A., "Motives for Drug Use: Adult and Adolescent," *Psychosomatics,* 13:317-324, 1972.

Fanshe, David, "Parental Failure and Consequences for Children," *American Journal of Public Health,* 65:604-612, June, 1975.

Goode, Erich, *The Marijuana Smokers,* New York: Basic Books, Publishers, 1970.

Grinspoon, Lester, "Marijuana," *Scientific American,* 221:17-26, December, 1969.

Heistad, Gordon, Martin Wong, and Robert Zimmerman, "Measuring Changes In Attitude Toward Drug Abuse: A Preliminary Report of a Method," *Journal of Drug Education,* 5:127-140, 1975.

**Hirschhorn, Kurt, 'LSD and Chromosomal Damage,"** *Hospital Practice,* 4:103, February, 1969.

Horowitz, Mardi J., "Flashback: Recurrent Intrusive Images after the Use of LSD," *American Journal of Psychiatry,* 126:147-151, October, 1969.

Julien, Robert, M., *A Primer of Drug Action,* San Francisco: W. H. Freeman and Company, 1975.

Louria, Donald, "A Critique of Some Current Approaches to the Problem of Drug Abuse," *American Journal of Public Health,* 65: 581-583, June, 1975.

McKee, Michael, "Drug Abuse Knowledge and Attitudes in 'Middle America,' " *American Journal of Public Health,* 65:584-590, June, 1975.

Means, Richard K., "Drug Abuse: Implications for Instruction," *JOHPER,* 41:22-24, 54, 55, May, 1970.

Nail, Richard L., "The Youthful Drug Abuser and Drug Abuse Education—Closing the Credibility Gap," *Journal of Drug Education,* 5:65-75, 1975.

Ray, Oakley S., *Drugs, Society and Human Behavior,* 2nd ed., St. Louis: Mosby, 1978.

Robinson, Paul E., "Beyond Drug Education," *Journal of Drug Education,* 5:183-191, 1975.

Schnoll, Sidney, "Poly Drug Abuse as Seen and Treated in a Free Clinic," *Journal of Psychodelic Drugs,* 7:229-236, April-June, 1975.

Sechrest, Dale, "Criminal Activity, Wages Earned, and Drug Use after Two Years of Methadone Treatment," *Addictive Diseases,* 1:491-512, 1975.

Singh, Mohan and Robert Steadward, "The Effects of Smoking Marijuana on Physical Performance," *Medicine and Science in Sports,* 7:309-311, Winter, 1975.

Smith, David, *The New Social Drug,* New Jersey: Prentice-Hall, 1970.

Smith, Mickey C., et al., "Kids, Drugs and the Druggist," *Journal of American Pharmaceutical Association,* 10:454-457, August, 1970.

## TEST QUESTIONS

### Multiple Choice Items

1. The two federal hospitals for the treatment of drug ad-

dicts are located in the states of: (a) New York and Georgia, (b) *Kentucky and Texas*, (c) Florida and New York, (d) California and New York, (e) Michigan and New York.

2. A person's reaction time when he is under the influence of a depressant becomes: (a) Increased, (b) *Decreased*, (c) Neither increased nor decreased, (d) Both increased and decreased, (e) None of the above.

3. Which statement is *not* true regarding amphetamines? (a) Benzedrine and dexedrine are example forms, (b) *They are classified as narcotics by present Federal law*, (c) Have a stimulating effect on the body, (d) Bennies is a slang term, (e) They are used medically for weight control.

4. Which statement is *not* true regarding barbiturates? (a) Nembutal and Amytal are examples, (b) They are useful to quiet disturbed or tense patients, (c) Physiological dependence occurs, (d) *Large doses are not fatal*, (e) They can be addictive.

5. Morphine has its primary effect upon which of the following? (a) Visual perception, (b) *Pain threshold*, (c) Auditory sense, (d) Gustatory sense, (e) All of the above.

6. Prescription-type sleeping pills contain the base of: (a) Marijuana, (b) Cocaine, (c) Heroin, (d) *Barbiturates*, (e) Benzedrine.

7. Which of the following is a resident house in California for the treatment of drug addicts? (a) LSD Rescue, (b) *Synanon*, (c) Narcotics Anonymous, (d) LeMar, (e) None of these.

8. Addiction to narcotic drugs is characterized by which of the following? (a) Habituation, (b) Tolerance, (c) Physical dependence, (d) None of these, (e) *All of these*.

9. Which of the following statements is *least* true of the amphetamine drugs? They: (a) Are legally sold by prescription, (b) Increase irritability and restlessness, (c) Interfere with the body's symptoms of fatigue, (d) *Have severe withdrawal symptoms worse than heroin*,

(e) Can cause body deterioration and complications more severe than heroin addiction.

10. The active ingredient in marijuana is identified by which of the following? (a) HTC, (b) CTH, (c) TCH, (d) MBT, (e) *THC.*

11. In the classification of drugs which of the following substances would be classified as a depressant? (a) Amphetamines, (b) LSD, (c) Peyote, (d) *Alcohol,* (e) Cocaine.

12. Physiological withdrawal would be expected from which of the following drugs? (a) Cocaine, (b) Marijuana, (c) *Morphine,* (d) LSD, (e) DMT.

13. Which of the following drugs is capable of producing sleep or stupor? (a) Amphetamine, (b) Benzedrine, (c) Cocaine, (d) *A narcotic,* (e) Mescal.

14. Which of the following best describes the presently known pharmacology of marijuana? (a) Harmless, (b) Well known, (c) *Poorly understood,* (d) The same as alcohol, (e) All of the above.

15. The medically prescribed drug considered to present the greatest total danger if abused is: (a) Marijuana, (b) Cocaine, (c) Heroin, (d) Tranquilizer, (e) *Barbiturates.*

16. The possibility of recovery from herion addiction today is: (a) *Very slight,* (b) Good for those who undergo treatment at a federal hospital, (c) Good for those who have a short history of addiction, (d) Improving greatly as more modern treatment is discovered, (e) Higher for males than for females.

17. A fatal dose of morphine or heroin causes death by depression of the vital processes of the: (a) Liver and kidney, (b) Heart, (c) Locomotion, (d) Respiratory system, (e) *Brain, respiratory system and heart.*

18. Which of the following senses is *mainly* affected while under the influence of LSD? (a) Auditory, (b) *Visual,* (c) Tactile, (d) Gustatory, (e) Smell.

19. The most severe withdrawal reaction results from ad-

diction to: (a) Marijuana, (b) Cocaine, (c) Heroin, (d) *Barbiturates*, (e) Mescaline.

20. Mescaline is derived from: (a) The Cocoa plant, (b) The Coca plant, (c) A poppy, (d) *A cactus*, (e) The Hemp plant.

## Matching Items

| | |
|---|---|
| 1. No legal use in the U.S. (d) | a. Morphine |
| 2. Ethyl (e) | b. Addiction |
| 3. Hallucinogen (f) | c. Chlorpromazine |
| 4. Amphetamine (i) | d. Heroin |
| 5. Opiate (a) or (d) | e. Beverage alcohol |
| 6. Psychological dependency (h) | f. Mescaline |
| | g. Antabuse |
| 7. Physical dependence (b) | h. Habituation |
| 8. Cannabis sativa (j) | i. Benzedrine |
| 9. Tranquilizer (c) | j. Marijuana |
| 10. Treatment for alcoholism (g) | k. None of these |

## Essay Items

1. A number of measures have been proposed and attempted in the control of drug addiction in the United States. What are some of the potential or existing measures that might be effective in the prevention or control of addiction?

2. Marijuana and heroin are classified in different drug categories. Briefly contrast the differences that exist between these two drugs with respect to their properties, influence, use, and other characteristics.

3. You learned of the availability on campus of amphetamines and that some students use them while studying for final examinations. Discuss some of the implications and ramifications of this practice as an adjustment mechanism.

4. A number of measures have been proposed and tried in the control of drug addiction in the United States.

What are five potential or existing measures that might be effective in the prevention or control of addiction?

5. Some drugs are distinctly classified as addicting, while others are more appropriately termed habit-forming. Indicate three common drugs that are normally construed to be habit-forming.

6. Using the extract below, and other information you have about the use of marijuana, answer the following questions.

*One more step is necessary if the user who has now learned to get high is to continue use. He must learn to enjoy the effects he has just learned to experience. Marijuana-produced sensations are not automatically or necessarily pleasurable. The taste for such experience is a socially acquired one, not different in kind from acquired tastes for oysters or dry martinis. The user feels dizzy, thirsty; his scalp tingles; he misjudges time and distances. Are these things pleasurable? He isn't sure. If he is to continue marijuana use, he must decide that they are. Otherwise, getting high, while a real enough experience, will be an unpleasant one he would rather avoid.*

*In short, what was once frightening and distasteful becomes, after a taste for it is built up, pleasant, desired, and sought after. Enjoyment is introduced by the favorable definition of the experience that one acquires from others. Without this, use will not continue, for marijuana will not be for the user an object he can use for pleasure.*

Source: Solomon, David, *The Marijuana Papers*, New York: Bobbs-Merrill Company, Inc., p. 42, 44.

a. What is the sequence of events and experiences by which a person comes to be able to carry on the use of marijuana in spite of the elaborate overt social controls functioning to prevent such behavior?

b. Since the "high" produced by marijuana is a "learned high" there is no justification perhaps for laws against the use of marijuana. Do you agree with this statement? Explain.

c. The above information seems to indicate that getting "high" is a conditioned response. If this is true, that there is no physical property of the plant which causes the "high," why is there so much furor over marijuana and why has it been used as an euphoria-producing drug for many centuries?

d. Explain what is meant by the term "socially acquired taste." Compare and contrast with the term "conditioning."

# SEXUALITY AND MARRIAGE

*Part Two* ❧ *Chapter* **14**

---

## BEHAVIORAL OBJECTIVES

The Student

- analyzes how human sexual identity develops

- summarizes the different ways in which the sexual drive can be expressed

- develops a personal code to guide sexual relationships

- distinguishes between how the early, agrarian, self-sufficient, cooperative family served its functions and how the modern-day family fulfills its purposes

- compares familial, economic, romantic, and other factors in mate selection

- discusses common marital adjustments that are necessary with all couples

# SUPPLEMENTARY TEACHING AIDS

*Phoebe: Story of a Premarital Pregnancy,* b / w, 28 min. This film depicts the mental and emotional reactions of a teen-age girl when she discovers she is pregnant. Alternate choices are presented for her to cope with this situation.

*The Game,* b / w, 28 min. The story of a teen-age girl and boy caught up in the dating game. Through open discussion the film provides the stimulus for reflection and discussion on double standard and premarital sex.

Both films are available from Contemporary Film, McGraw-Hill, 828 Custer Ave., Evanston, Ill., 60202.

*Homosexuality: What About McBride?* Popular stereotypes of sexual behavior create patterns of interpersonal relations. Social isolation may be forced on individuals because of doubts about sexual behavior. This film presents a realistic situation of young people questioning who in their group might be a homosexual. CRM Educational Films, Del Mar, Calif. 92014.

*Women Who Have Had an Abortion,* Women of all ages, races and socio-economic levels explain their search for and experiences in obtaining an abortion. The open candor and personal experience reputes stereotyped images of women who seek abortion. Martha Stuart Communications, 66 Bank Street, New York, N.Y. 10014.

*On Being An Effective Parent,* The no-lose method of parental guidance is explained by Dr. Thomas Gordon. Skills of active listening and accurate communication of feelings are demonstrated in role-playing situations. 2 reels, $30.00 / day rental fee. American Personnel and Guidance Association, Film Department, 1607 New Hampshire Ave. N.W., Washington, D.C. 20009.

The following three films on sexuality and sexual expression are excellent for classroom discussion.

*Like Other People.* A very moving story of two young people with physical handicaps and their quality of life and marriage.

*Value.* The personal story of a drag queen and her transition into a different life style. Her family's reaction and treatment attempts are explored. The purpose of the film is not to shock and ridicule, but to understand the range of possible human sexual expression.

*Lavender.* The private thoughts and feelings of two young women are explored through flash backs of their childhood. Their acceptance of their homosexual society is questioned. The concept of love is presented as human expression in heterosexual and homosexual forms. Perennial Education, Inc., 1625 Willow Road, Northfield, Illinois 60093.

Request film listing from: Population Dynamics, 3829 Aurora Ave. N., Seattle, Washington 98103.

*Beyond Conception,* color, 35 min. A comprehensive film that explains the threat of over-population and available medical means of birth control. The methods of birth control are presented with factors that influence personal decisions regarding selection of a personal birth control procedure. Population Dynamics, 3829 Aurora Ave. N., Seattle, Washington 98103.

## Filmstrips

*Parenting Education, Child Abuse, Death.* Write to Parents' Magazine Films, Inc., 52 Vanderbilt Ave., New York, N.Y. 10017 for filmstrip descriptive flyers.

This is a good source for up-to-date filmstrips on child abuse, death, divorce and separation, illness and its effect on children.

## ORGANIZATIONS THAT HAVE MATERIALS *

American Association of Marriage and Family, 2257 Yale Ave., Claremont, Calif. 91711.

American Association of Sex Educators and Counselors, 815 15th St., N.W., Washington, D.C. 20005.

American Home Economics Association, 2010 Massachusetts Ave., N. W., Washington, D. C. 20036.

American Institute of Family Relations, Inc., 5287 Sunset Blvd., Los Angeles, Calif. 90027.

Educational Foundation for Human Sexuality, Montclair State College, Upper Montclair, N. J. 07043.

Institute for Family Research and Education, 760 Ostrom Ave., Syracuse, N. Y. 13210.

Institute for Sex Research, Inc., Room 416, Morrison Hall, Indiana University, Bloomington, Ind. 47401.

National Council on Family Relations, 1219 University Ave., S.E., Minneapolis, Minn. 55414.

National Foundation — March of Dimes, 275 Mamaroneck Ave., Box 2000, White Plains, N. Y. 10602.

National Institute of Child Health and Human Development, Room

2a-03, Building 31, 900 Rockville Pike, Bethesda, Md. 20015.

National Organization for Non-Parents, 806 Reisertown Rd., Baltimore, Md. 21208.

National Parents & Teachers Association, 1425 H St., N. W., Washington, D. C. 20005.

National Right to Life, Inc., National Press Building, 529 14th St., N. W., Washington, D. C. 20045.

Parenting Materials Information Center, Southwest Education Development Lab, 211 East 7th St., Austin, Tx. 78701.

Parents Without Partners, 7910 Woodmont Ave., Bethesda, Md. 20014.

Sex Information and Education Council of the U.S., 1855 Broadway, New York, N.Y. 10023.

Tampax, Inc., Department IRM, P.O. Box 7001, Lake Success, N. Y. 11040.

*The addresses of these organizations and their policies concerning the sending of materials are subject to change without notice.*

## STUDENT INVOLVEMENT

### Investigations

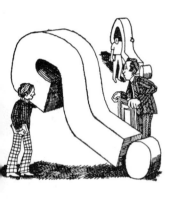

Describe how the so-called double standard affects dating practices and mate selection.

What are the factors in teen-age marriages that contribute to greater failures than in marriages at older ages?

What types of adjustive problems might the widow or widower expect?

What is the role in society for the single person? Can a single person find happiness in a couple-oriented culture?

Describe the common fallacies and superstitions espoused about masturbation. Where did these ideas originate?

Debate the pros and cons of prescribing birth control pills for unmarried women. How has this practice affected the rate of venereal disease and other genital tract infections?

Is homosexuality a condition, a problem, a disease? Discuss various views.

Determine the laws in the state regulating the practice of marriage counselors. Is there licensing, a registry, etc.?

Make a directory of resources available in your home community for premarital and marital counseling services.

Write a short essay on what marital love means to me. Use these essays as a basis for class discussion on this topic.

What role in society is allowed to divorced individuals? What special problems confront them?

Review smoking advertisements over the past thirty-five years to study society's attitude toward women and smoking.

What alternate life styles are being tried today? Make a study of communes, group marriages, etc.

What is meant by the term *free love?*

Has the pill changed the concept of morality?

Trace the history of women's rights in the United States. Is the current women's liberation movement a new concept?

Study television commercials. What concept of women and their role in society is presented. Do commercials exploit women as the women's lib people insist?

Discuss the concept of unisex. What does it mean? Is it just a dress fad?

## Action

Display advertising materials that illustrate the exploitation of sex to sell a product.

Interview students on their views of the Women's Liberation Movement and on the Gay Liberation Movement.

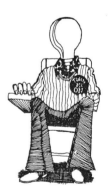

Survey students on their opinions of the value of Sex Education and Family Life Courses. What do they believe should be the objectives and topics, and who should teach the courses?

Survey married students on the pros and cons of marriage while in college. What problems do they have that cause the most difficulties in their marriage?

Survey older students on campus on their attitudes toward sexuality and contrast this with the attitudes held by the younger students. Is there that much difference, and if so, in what areas? Also, what factors were most influential in shaping their attitudes?

Interview married people on the problems faced in their marriage. What areas seem to cause the most difficulties in the marriages and what are some solutions to these common problems?

Interview a local physician on the pros and cons of the pill.

Present a class discussion on some ideas of alternate life styles in family living.

## BASIC SOURCE MATERIALS

Arnstein, Robert L., "Anxiety About Homosexuality," *Human Sexuality*, 10:189-90, January, 1976.

Aurbach, Aline B., "Parents' Role in Day Care," *Child Care Quarterly*, 4:180-86, Fall, 1975.

Beach, Frank, "It's All in Your Mind," *Psychology Today*, 3:33-35, 60, July, 1969.

Beasley, Ruth, "Current Status of Sex Research," *The Journal of Sex Research*, 11:335-47, November, 1975.

Coummette, Beauty, "Transitions in Motherhood," *Maternal — Child Nursing Journal*, 4:65-73, Summer, 1975.

Cvetkovich, George, et al., "On the Psychology of Adolescents' Use of Contraceptives," *The Journal of Sex Research*, 11:256-70, August, 1975.

Eastman, William, et al., "Viewpoint: How Do Young People Usually React to Their First Intercourse?" *Human Sexuality*, 10:32-42, January, 1976.

Feeley, Ellen, and Helen Pyne, "The Menopause: Facts and Misconceptions," *Nursing Forum*, 14:74-86, 1975.

Finger, Frank W., "Changes in Sex Practices and Beliefs of Male College Students During 30 Years," *The Journal of Sex Research*, 11:304-17, November, 1975.

Fromme, Alan, *The Ability to Love,* California: Borden Publishing Co., 1966.

Gagnon, John, H., and William Simon, "They Are Going to Learn in the Street Anyway," *Psychology Today*, 3:48-49, 71, July, 1969.

"Gays on the March," *Time*, 106:10, 32-37, September 8, 1975.

Gilberg, Arnold, "The Stress of Parenting," *Child Psychiatry and Human Development*, 6:59-67, Winter, 1975.

Goodheart, Barbara, "Education on Titillation," *Today's Health*, 48:28-30, 70, February, 1970.

Greenberg, Martin, and Norman Morris, "Engrossment: The Newborn's Impact Upon the Father," *Nursing Digest,* 4:19-22, January/February, 1976.

Heiman, Julia R. "Women's Sexual Arousal," *Psychology Today,* 91-94, April, 1975.

Kaye, Elizabeth, "Falling in Love May Be Hazardous to Your Health," *Family Health,* 10:22-25, March, 1978.

Kessler, Sheila, "Divorce Adjustment Groups," *The Personnel and Guidance Journal,* 54:250-55, January, 1976.

Kriegman, George, "Homosexuality and the Educator," *Journal of School Health,* 39:305-311, May, 1969.

Maguire, Daniel, "The Vatican on Sex," *Commonweal,* 103:137-140, February, 1976.

Marquart, Roberta, "Expectant Fathers: What Are Their Needs?" *Maternal — Child Nursing Journal,* 1:32-36, January/February, 1976.

Masters, William H., and Virginia E. Johnson, *Human Sexual Inadequacy,* Boston: Little, Brown and Co., 1970.

Murray, Linda, "Sexual Boredom: What It Means in a Relationship," *Family Health,* 9:22-26, June, 1977.

Nichols, Beverly, "The Abused Wife Problem," *Social Casework,* 57:27-32, January, 1976.

"Playboy Interview: Dr. Mary Calderone," *Playboy,* 14:63-78, April, 1970.

Runciman, Alexander, "Sexual Therapy of Masters and Johnson," *The Counseling Psychologist,* 5:22-30, 1975.

Sheely, Gail, Gloria Steinem, Pete Hamil, "Love in the Age of Options," *New York,* 3:28-52, February 16, 1970.

Van Dusen, Roxann, and Eleanor Sheldon, "The Changing Status of American Women," *American Psychologist,* 31:106-116, February, 1976.

"Why So Many Wives Are Running Away," *U.S. News and World Report,* 80:24-25, February, 1976.

Young, Christabel M., "Factors Associated with Timing and Duration of Leaving-Home Stage of the Family Life Cycle," *Population Studies,* 29:61-73, March, 1975.

# TEST QUESTIONS

## Multiple Choice Items

1. In discussing sex roles a valid premise is that: (a) One sex is superior to the other, (b) Feminine and masculine

roles are quite well defined, (c) Sex roles have not really changed much during this century, (d) *Sex roles are currently in a state of flux*, (e) Sex makes no difference to role expectation.

2. Much of the difficulty in marital adjustment might be attributed to: (a) The emancipation of women, (b) Economic independence of women, (c) *Differences in belief about the role of husband and wife*, (d) Lack of a well defined authority head in the family, (e) In-law relationships.

3. The principal deterrent to premarital sex relations appears to be: (a) The fear of pregnancy, (b) Fear of contracting a venereal disease, (c) *Conceptions of morality*, (d) Concern about one's reputation, (e) Regard for the partner.

4. The matter of sexual adjustment in marriage is primarily: (a) Biological, (b) *Psychological*, (c) Cultural, (d) Anatomical, (e) Social.

5. The basic reason for getting married today is: (a) To avoid getting drafted, (b) *For love and companionship*, (c) To live a longer life, (d) Parental pressure, (e) To escape tyrannical parents.

6. The age at time of first marriage for half of the people in the United States is: (a) *21 and below for females, 23 or below for males*, (b) 18 for both males and females, (c) 18 for females, 25 for males, (d) 24 for females, 27 for males, (e) Over 21 for both male and female.

7. A person's readiness for marriage is best evaluated in terms of many important factors. From among the following, the most important factor is probably: (a) Sexual maturity, (b) Economic capacity, (c) *Emotional maturity*, (d) Social responsibility, (e) Intelligence.

8. Successful adjustment in marriage is probably most dependent upon: (a) Conformity to a pattern established by the husband, (b) Adherence to plans developed by the wife, (c) The realization that sex is the only vital

part of marriage, (d) The management of finances by the wife, (e) *Working together toward worthwhile goals.*

9. Which will tend to help a marriage be successful? (a) The husband helps with the housework, (b) *Personal attractiveness is maintained,* (c) The wife has one night out, (d) The husband takes care of all finances, (e) The wife works.

10. Second marriages are what percent more risky than first: (a) Ten percent, (b) Twenty percent, (c) Thirty percent, (d) Forty percent, (e) *Fifty percent.*

11. In selecting a marriage partner, it is proven wisest to: (a) Have the parents make the selection, (b) *Use the head as well as the heart,* (c) Give first consideration to economic status, (d) Consider social background of primary importance, (e) Choose on the basis of physical appearance.

12. Among the following, the factor which best assures successful marriage for a couple is that they: (a) Both like children, (b) Both like the same things, (c) Both are willing to work and sacrifice for a home, (d) *Both come from happy, well-adjusted homes,* (e) Have had about the same amount of education.

13. Those anticipating marriage should be aware of possible problem situations. According to reliable authorities, the two areas of probably greatest adjustment in marriage are: (a) *Spending family income and sex relations,* (b) Personal mannerisms and in-law relations, (c) Smoking and social activities, (d) Mutual friends and untidiness, (e) Drinking and bossiness.

14. The characteristics of romantic love feelings of elation, depression and anxiety (a) Are signs of true love, (b) Happen only once in a life time, (c) Are indications of the compatibility of the couple, (d) Are an accurate indication that there is depth in the relationship at the time, (e) *Are probably a reflection of emotional instability of the relationship at the time.*

15. The studies of steady dating indicate that the percentage of people dating steadily and the number of persons dated: (a) Has changed markedly in the present generation, (b) Has not changed markedly in the present generation, (c) Is a factor contributing to

unhappiness in marriage, (d) *Has probably not changed significantly over the past 30 years,* (e) Has no significance to marital happiness.

16. Trial marriages by college students: (a) Is a new 1970s arrangement, (b) *Is an arrangement that has existed on college campuses for years,* (c) Hardly ever results in marriage, (d) Involves no committment, (e) Is a declining practice.

17. In a mature love relationship: (a) It is inevitable that one partner will emerge as the dominating personality, (b) Individuality cannot be maintained, (c) *There is no need for control or domination of one by the other,* (d) There is a guarantee of agreement in all phases of life, (e) The female will be dominant.

18. "Love at first sight": (a) Is best described as true love, (b) *Can be confused with emotional excitement created by sexual attraction to a nice-looking person,* (c) Cannot be developed into a deeper relationship since the foundation is a sexual attraction, (d) Cannot be explained, (e) Is a myth and never occurs.

19. Important changes occurred in the structure of the American family: (a) During the Westward movement, the Industrial era and Emancipation of women, (b) During the Westward movement, the Emancipation of women and World War II, (c) *During the Westward movement, the Industrial era and World Wars I and II,* (d) During the Emancipation of women and after World War II, (e) After World Wars I and II.

20. Studies on the relationship of premarital sexual experience to marital adjustments indicate: (a) Better adjustment in marriage, (b) More difficult adjustment in marriage, (c) *Neither more positive nor more difficult adjustment in marriage,* (d) That premarital experience is more advisable for males than females, (e) That premarital experience contributes to better adjustment for females with positive attitudes towards sex.

## Matching Items

1. Most important factor in mate selection (d)
2. Compatibility and com-

   a. Love
   b. Marriage
   c. Happiness and success

mon interests (g)
3. Intimate behavior (c)
4. Important adjustment in marriage (f)
5. Phenomenon (h)
6. Concern of two people for each other (a)
7. Cooperation (c)
8. Companionship, affection, satisfaction (b)
9. Social practice (j)
10. Means of problem solving (e)

d. Dependable character
e. Divorce
f. Sex
g. Engagement
h. Love at first sight
i. Petting
j. Dating

## Essay Items

1. What are some of the factors that should be considered in deciding whether or not to marry a particular person?

2. The nature of family life in the United States has changed in the last fifty years. Indicate some of these changes by contrast with past generations. What factors have led to these changes? What present factors or future events might change family life in the next twenty-five years?

3. List some of the characteristics of a good wife or husband. Which are most important to you?

4. What are some of the necessary areas of adjustment after marriage? How might they be resolved? What are adjustments for the new husband, the new wife?

5. Discuss the purposes and relationships of dating, going steady, getting pinned and becoming engaged. Are these rituals outdated today?

6. Using the following concept of Sex Education, discussions from class, and your own ideas of the objectives of Sex Education, present your ideas on the real objectives of Sex Education. You may list in order of importance. This refers to general goals that would apply to any age level.

*Sex educators and sexologists now talk about human sexuality rather than sex. Sex, connoting anatomical*

*difference, physiological process, or the sex act, is
too limited a concept. In the foreword to a syllabus for
Family Life Education from kindergarten through high
school, Don Cannaday, Assistant Director of the
Family Health Association of Cleveland, writes: "By
sexuality I mean the whole gamut of being males and
females in any kind of relationship. This includes, of
course, the whole puzzling richness of masculine-
feminine dimensions."*

*Mr. Cannaday holds that it is no longer realistic or
desirable to have sex control as our primary goal in
Sex Education. "However important control may be
in certain temporary situations," he says, "it is not a
big enough goal, nor is it one worthy of our best
energy. Neither can our goal for human sexuality be
the kind of casual, carefree, playboy abandon that
some would advocate. . . . Somewhere between rigid,
repressive and moralistic control and loose,
irresponsible abandon there is what I have chosen to
call the celebration of sexuality, and this is what we
must strive for." By "celebration," Mr. Cannaday
says he means "not any one specific act, but a
continuing positive and joyful acceptance of being
sexual, and the concern to experience this and express
it in ways that will be most beneficial for the individual
and the community."*

7. Organize a chart to outline your thoughts on what concepts of sexuality should be taught at the various age
levels and suggested ways in which the concept may
be presented. Divide the age levels as follows:

| Grade | Concept | Ways to Present | Who Should Present |
|-------|---------|-----------------|--------------------|
| K-3 | | | |
| 4-6 | | | |
| 7-9 | | | |
| 10-12 | | | |
| College | | | |

# REPRODUCTION AND FAMILY PLANNING

*Part Two* e3 *Chapter 15*

---

## BEHAVIORAL OBJECTIVES

The Student

- demonstrates knowledge of the physiological aspects of the reproductive process

- selects appropriate methods for spacing pregnancies

- identifies the relationships between prenatal care and the healthy child

- understands the mechanism of childbirth physically and emotionally

- distinguishes facts from myths and superstition surrounding human reproduction and childbirth

# SUPPLEMENTARY TEACHING AIDS

*An Unfinished Story*, 13½ min. A dramatic film about a young mother with three children who feels that her family's future will be threatened by the birth of another child. She seeks the counsel of her minister, a lawyer and her doctor. A friend tells her about legal abortions abroad. Her search for a dignified, safe solution to this problem breaks off at the point of decision regarding an illegal abortion — leaving the story and society's response to this problem unfinished. Association for the Study of Abortion, Inc., 120 West 57th St., New York, N.Y. 10019.

*First Two Weeks of Life*, color, 17 min. This film is a tender, but realistic narrative of a baby and its arrival in the world. Prepared childbirth and the physical changes of an infant during the first few weeks of life are explained. Association-Sterling Films, 600 Grand Avenue, Ridgefield, N. J. 07657.

*A Mother's Wish*, color, 13 min. What kind of world awaits future children? Can we guarantee them a healthy and safe world? This film presents a young mother's hopes and wishes for her infant. Association-Sterling Films, 600 Grand Avenue, Ridgefield, N. J. 07657.

*Newborn*, color, 28 min. The development of an infant in the first three months of life is presented in this joyful film. The basic questions of how to care for a newborn are answered. Because so many young people have had no experience with caring for infants, this film is immensely valuable for health classes. The fears of new parents are addressed in a reassuring manner. Association-Sterling Films, 600 Grand Avenue, Ridgefield, N. J. 07657.

Request special up-to-date materials from the National Foundation — March of Dimes, local chapters or National Headquarters, 1275 Mamaroneck Avenue, White Plains, N. Y. 10602. (films, filmstrips, exhibits, pamphlets).

REQUEST FILM CATALOG from Planned Parenthood-World Population, Film Library, 810 Seventh Ave., New York, N. Y. 10019 (clinical and general audience films).

Transparency Originals (See Part 3 of Handbook)

## ORGANIZATIONS THAT HAVE MATERIALS *

American Academy of Pediatrics, 1801 Hinson Ave., Evanston, Ill. 60204.

American Medical Association, Bureau of Health Education, 535 N. Dearborn St., Chicago, Ill. 60610.

American Institute of Family Relations, 5287 Sunset Boulevard, Los Angeles, Calif. 90027.

Association for Voluntary Sterilization, 708 Third Ave., New York, N. Y. 10017.

Child Study Association of America, 15 Madison Ave., New York, N. Y. 10019.

Center for Medical Consumers, 55 Washington Square South, New York, N. Y. 10003.

Family Service Association of America, 44 East 23rd St., New York, N. Y. 10017.

Institute for Sex Research, Inc., Room 416, Morrison Hall, Indiana University, Bloomington, Ind. 47401.

Johnson and Johnson, 501 George St., New Brunswick, N. J. 08901.

Kimberly-Clark Corporation, Educational Service, Neenah, Wis., 54956.

National Center for Family Planning Services, 5600 Fishers Lane, Rockville, Md. 20852.

National Congress of Parents and Teachers, 700 N. Rush St., Chicago, Ill. 60611.

National Genetics Foundation, Inc., 250 W. 57th St., New York, N. Y. 10019.

Personal Products Corporation, Educational Department, Milltown, N. J. 08850.

Planned Parenthood Federation of America, 545 Madison Ave., New York, N. Y. 10022.

Population Association of America, 806 15th St., N. W., Washington, D. C. 20005.

Population Institution, 110 Maryland Ave., N. E., Washington, D. C. 20002.

Public Affairs Committee, Inc., 381 Park Ave. S., New York, N. Y. 10016.

Tampax, Inc., Department IRM, P.O. Box 7001, Lake Success, N. Y. 11040.

*The addresses to these organizations and their policies concerning the sending of materials are subject to change without notice.*

## STUDENT INVOLVEMENT

### Investigations

How can the working mother assure that the emotional needs of her child will be met?

What are the advantages and disadvantages of natural childbirth? Birth under anesthesia and the various positions / delivery?

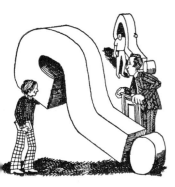

How do exercises for birth aid labor?

What are the major types of congenital anomalies? How can their incidence be reduced? What are some legal and moral questions involved with genetic counseling, "human engineering"? Where are genetic counseling services available? Contact the National Foundation.

How dangerous is the Rh factor? Caesarian birth?

What are some inherited defects that seem to be racially determined?

What organizations offer prenatal classes in the community?

What is the La Leche League and is there such a group in your area?

What are the pros and cons of breast feeding, and the relationship to breast cancer?

Compare hospitalization costs to have a baby and costs covered by Health Insurance.

What factors contribute to such a high infant mortality rate in the U.S.?

What is the latest information regarding proper weight gain during pregnancy?

What does recent research indicate is the relationship between prenatal nutrition and the development of the infant brain and subsequent intelligence?

What factors have contributed to the increased popularity of delivery by a mid-wife?

### Action

What day care facilities are available or should be available in your community? Make a survey.

Visit prenatal care classes sponsored by the local Red Cross or hospital clinic. Report on observations.

What special foods are available through food stamps for

pregnant women? Visit the local U.S.D.A. Extension Office or the Welfare Department and assess the value of this program. Is the food packaged in easy-to-carry packages? Are the available services utilized?

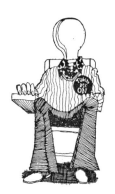

Contact the local National Foundation-March of Dimes and volunteer for the College Action Program in Prenatal Care Education and Service Project.

Conduct interviews of social workers at agencies that place children for adoption. What are some problems encountered in finding good homes for adoptive children?

Survey attitudes among college students as to size of family desired. What seems to be the ideal family size? How is this decision derived? Are young, child-bearing age men and women conscious of the population explosion? Is this a reality in their individual decision making or only an intellectual awareness?

Visit a Birth Defect Treatment Center of the National Foundation-March of Dimes. Request permission to observe or interview parents on the problems involved in loving and caring for a child with congenital problems.

Visit, or correspond with several communes that are experimenting with alternate family life styles. Report on observations.

## BASIC SOURCE MATERIALS

Abernethy, Virginia and Henry Grunebaum, "Marital Decision-Making As Applied to Family Planning," *Journal of Sex & Marital Therapy*, I:63-73, Fall, 1974.

Barnes, S., Eugene and Stuart Fors, "Who Are Wednesday's Children?" *Journal of School Health*, 46:37-39, January, 1976.

Brinley, Maryann B., "Crucial Questions of an Expectant Mother," *Family Health*, 10:8, 10, 46, May 1978.

Green, Lawrence, Andrew Fisher, Ruhul Amin and A. Shafmillah, "Path To the Adoption of Family Planning," *International Journal of Health Education*, 18:85-96, April/June, 1975.

"Having a Baby—A Complete Guide to the Latest in Maternity Care," *Family Health*, 7:35-38, 40-46, October, 1975.

Herbeneck, Raymond M., "Remarks on Abortion, Abandonment and Adoption Opportunities," *Philosophy and Public Affairs*, 5:98-104, Fall, 1975.

Houde, Charlotte et al., "Teen-Age Mothers: A Clinical Profile," *Contemporary Ob/Gyn*, 7:71-78, January, 1976.

Irwin, Theodore, "Birth Order—What it Means to Your Children," *Today's Health*, 47:26-27, 79-80, 84-86, October, 1969.

Katz, Barbara J., "The IUD: Out of Sight, Out of Mind?" *Ms.* 4:108-110, 113-115, July, 1975.

Luy, Mary, "The Male Pill—Knotty Problem or Misogynist Myth?" *Modern Medicine*, 43, 42-46, October, 1975.

Lyon, Fred, "The Development of Adenocarcinoma of the Endometrium in Young Women Receiving Long Term Sequental Oral Contraception," *Obstetrical and Gynecological Survey*, 31:219-222, March, 1976.

MacCorquodale, Donald, "A Study of the Effectiveness of Family Planning Clinics in the Philippines," *Public Health Reports*, 90:490-497, November/December, 1975.

Machol, Libby, "Birth Control: Which Way Is Best?" *Family Health*, 8:34-36, 66, 68, 70, 72, April 1977.

Michol, Libby, and Paul T. Wilson, "Abortion—The Medical Facts," *Family Health*, 8:42-45, 60, February, 1976.

Needle, Richard H., "Factors Affecting Contraceptive Practices of High School and College-Age Students," *Journal of School Health*, 47:340-45, June, 1977.

Peterson, James A., *Love in the Later Years*, New York: Association Press, 1975.

Porter, Cedric W. and Jaroslav F. Hulka, "Female Sterilization in Current Clinical Practice," *Family Planning Perspectives*, 6:8-15, Winter, 1974.

Qadeer, Mohammed A., "Why Family Planning is Failing," *Social Policy*, 6:19-23, November/December, 1975.

Quent, Barbara, "Seven Mistakes Women Make with Money," *Money*, 4:61-62, December, 1975.

"Solving the Contraceptive Conundrum," *Moneysworth*, 12-13, July 21, 1975.

Sorley, Anne, "Prescribing a Contraceptive Method," *The Nurse Practitioner, A Journal of Primary Nursing Care*, 1:55-59, November/December, 1975.

Thompson, Judi, "Expecting—The Yogo Way," *Family Health*, 10:44-46, March, 1978.

Trotter, Robert J., "Changing the Face of Birth," *Science News*, 108:9, 106-108, August 16, 1975.

"Vasectomy Reversal That Really Works," *Medical World News*, 16:19-21, November 17, 1975.

Weidger, Paul, "Diaphragms, A New Look At the Old Standby," *Ms.* 4:108-110, July, 1975.

## TEST QUESTIONS

### Multiple Choice Items

1. Collectively male hormones are known as: (a) Estrogens, (b) Semen, (c) *Androgens*, (d) Deferens, (e) Epididymis.

2. The uterus is part of the: (a) Male reproductive system, (b) *Female reproductive system*, (c) Embryo, (d) Excretory system, (e) Urinary system.

3. All of the following are part of the female reproductive system, except: (a) Gonads, (b) Fallopian tubes, (c) Uterus, (d) Cervix, (e) *Prostate.*

4. Which of the following statements is *least* true regarding multiple births? (a) There have been no substantiated cases of six or more children born to a human, (b) Fraternal twins are more frequent than identical twins, (c) Identical twins are always of the same sex, (d) Siamese twins are identical twins that have not completely separated, (e) *Fraternal twins result from the fertilization of a single ovum.*

5. Which is not a fallacy about menstruation? (a) It is bad to stop or shorten a period because the poisons cannot get out, (b) Sitting in warm water will start or stop a period, (c) Women are unclean during menstruation, (d) *During a menstrual period a woman will feel comfortable if she bathes frequently,* (e) Sexual relations during menstruation are harmful.

6. The gamete contains the following number of chromosomes: (a) None, (b) *Twenty-three*, (c) Forty-six, (d) Ninety-two, (e) Forty-eight.

7. The most successful method of preventing conception has been the: (a) *Pill*, (b) Diaphragm, (c) Condom, (d) Rhythm method, (e) Douche.

8. Spermatozoa arise from cells located in the: (a) *Testes*, (b) Fallopian tubes, (c) Uterus, (d) Ureter, (e) Prostate gland.

9. All inherited characteristics of new life are determined: (a) *Immediately when one sperm penetrates the ovum in the Fallopian tube*, (b) Six to twelve hours after this union, (c) During the first twenty-four hours after fertilization, (d) Sometime during the first week of pregnancy, (e) During the first seventy-two hours following fertilization.

10. Fertilization of the ovum by the sperm occurs normally in: (a) The vagina, (b) The cervix, (c) The uterus, (d) *The Fallopian tube*, (e) The Ovary.

11. Which is not an old wives tale about pregnancy? (a) Bathing is dangerous, (b) Exercise will cause a miscarriage, (c) *Excessive weight aggravates discomforts*, (d) Sex relations are hazardous, (e) A fall or blow will bring on a miscarriage.

12. The release of the female reproductive cell from the ovary is a process known as: (a) Menstruation, (b) Gestation, (c) *Ovulation*, (d) Menopause, (e) Fertilization.

13. If fertilized, the ovum implants itself on the: (a) Cervix, (b) *Uterine wall*, (c) Vagina, (d) Hymen, (e) Labium majora.

14. What period of embryonic development is the most crucial: (a) Two to four weeks, (b) *Four to six weeks*, (c) Six to eight weeks, (d) Eight to ten weeks, (e) Ten to twelve weeks.

15. Ovulation in the human female usually occurs: (a) Two weeks after menstruation, (b) During menstruation, (c) Halfway between menstrual periods, (d) *Two weeks before menstruation*, (e) Several days following menstruation.

16. The bag of waters in which the fetus develops is called the: (a) Placenta, (b) Scrotal sac, (c) *Amniotic sac*, (d) Bladder, (e) Umbilical sac.

17. The trigger that sets off the process of labor is: (a) The size of the fetus, (b) *Not exactly known*, (c) The length of gestation, (d) The weight of the fetus, (e) The amount of estrogen in the fetus.

18. When a woman thinks she is probably pregnant, after

a missed period, she should: (a) Increase her amount of sleep, (b) *Be examined by a physician*, (c) Increase her food intake, (d) Stop working, (e) Take the pill.

19. The discharge from the vagina during menstruation is composed of: (a) The unfertilized ovum, (b) Blood and lining cells from the ovary, (d) Waste material from the genitourinary tract, (d) *Blood and lining cells from the uterus*, (e) Hormone secretions.

20. Any woman during the childbearing years should assume she is pregnant if following intercourse she: (a) *Misses one menstrual period*, (b) Misses two menstrual periods, (c) Has increased urination, (d) Has a lump in her breast, (e) Feels fatigued.

## Matching Items

1. Another name for uterus (c)
2. Device to prevent pregnancy (e)
3. Temporary period when conception cannot occur (i)
4. Female (h)
5. Mechanism of excreting sperm (b)
6. Male (j)
7. Pains of childbirth (d)
8. Location of the testes (a)
9. Inability to fertilize (f)
10. Birth canal (g)

a. Scrotum
b. Ejaculation
c. Womb
d. Labor
e. Contraceptive
f. Sterility
g. Vagina
h. Chromosome X
i. Infertility
j. Chromosome Y
k. None of these

## Essay Items.

1. What emotional and physiological difficulties do women sometimes experience with the onset of menopause?

2. How does good prenatal care help make childbirth safer for both mother and child?

3. Describe the stages of labor in childbirth.

4. Discuss the moral, social and medical issues of abortion.

5. What social and moral issues might be involved in deciding the number of children a couple wishes to have?

# DEBILITATORS: CHRONIC AND DEGENERATIVE DISEASES

*Part Two* ℰ *Chapter* **16**

---

## BEHAVIORAL OBJECTIVES

The Student

- identifies the chronic and degenerative diseases that un-necessarily deprive individuals of happy, productive years of life

- recognizes early symptoms of chronic and degenerative conditions to obtain early medical supervision

- has periodical medical examinations that are a major health practice that reduce the incidence of, retards the effects of, and prevents premature death from, the de-bilitators

- maintains personal medical records

- evaluates the constituents of good preventive health care

- is informed of the nature of some of the more common diseases and disorders to reduce susceptibility to quackery

# SUPPLEMENTARY TEACHING AIDS

*The Heart: Attack,* color, 27 min. This film effectively demonstrates the results of the combined effects of years of heart attack risk factors. Each factor is examined and possible risk reduction actions are explained. The Framingham Study. CRM Educational Films, Del Mar, Calif. 92014.

*The Heart: Counterattack,* Prevention is presented as the main offensive against a heart attack. Simple but direct cause/effect relationships of cigarette smoking, weight, exercise and stress are demonstrated. The film shows how people can assess their risk and take steps to lessen their vulnerability. CRM Educational Films, Del Mar, Calif. 92014.

*Looking at Children,* color, 24 min. This film presents a documentary of actual case histories of chronic and communicable diseases in young children. Designed to prepare teachers to identify signs of illness in children. Also may be useful in college health classes. Metropolitan Life Insurance, Health and Welfare Division, One Madison Avenue, New York, N. Y. 10010.

*Progress Against Cancer,* color, 28 min. Cancer is probably the most mysterious and feared disease today. Extensive research in the last decade has provided cures never dreamed possible. Well known T.V. and screen stars tell intimate stories of fights against cancer. The film intends to enlighten and relieve the fears of cancer. Association-Sterling Films, 600 Grand Avenue, Ridgefield, N. J. 07657.

*Research to Prevent Cancer,* color, 18 min. Researchers and famous T.V. personalities explain the progress in treating cancer. Emphasis is placed on the improving survival rate. This film is biologically oriented with some in-depth interviews with physicians. Association-Sterling Films, 600 Grand Avenue, Ridgefield, N. J. 07657.

*Second Chance to Live,* color, 28 min. This film demonstrates how combined efforts by a community to protect itself saves lives. Seattle, Washington has combined public health education with a well trained crew of emergency medical technicians. All communities are urged to organize such a program. Metropolitan Life Insurance, Health and Welfare Divison, One Madison Avenue, New York, N.Y. 10010.

Contact your local American Lung Association and American Cancer Society for Current film catalogs.

Transparency Originals (See Part 3 of Handbook)

## ORGANIZATIONS THAT HAVE MATERIALS *

American Cancer Society, Inc., 319 East 42nd St., New York, N.Y. 10017.

American Diabetes Association, Inc., 18 E. 48th St., New York, N.Y. 10017.

Allergy Foundation of America, 801 2nd Ave., New York, N. Y. 10017.

Arthritis Foundation, 1212 Ave. of the Americas, New York, N.Y. 10036.

The American Health Foundation, Inc., 180 East End Ave., New York, N.Y. 10028.

American Heart Association, Inquiries Section, 44 E. 23rd St., New York, N. Y. 10010.

American Lung Association, 1740 Broadway, New York, N. Y. 10019.

American Public Health Association, 1015 18th St., N. W., Washington, D. C. 20036.

Center for Disease Control, 1600 Clifton Rd., N. E., Atlanta, Ga. 30333.

Epilepsy Foundation, 1828 L St., N. W., Washington, D. C. 20036.

Leukemia Society, Inc., 211 E. 43rd St., New York, N.Y. 10017.

The National Council on the Aging, 1825 L Street, N. W., Suite 501, Washington, D. C. 20036.

National Cystic Fibrosis Research Foundation, 202 E. 44th St., N.Y. 10017.

National Epilepsy League, Inc., 203 N. Wabash St., Chicago, Ill. 60601.

National Foundation for Ileitis and Colitis, 295 Madison Ave., New York, N. Y. 10017.

National Foundation for Neuro-Muscular Diseases, 250 W. 57th St., New York, N.Y. 10019.

National Hemophilia Foundation, 25 W. 37th St., New York, N.Y. 10018.

National Institute of Arthritis, Metabolism and Digestive Disorders, Room 9A-52, Building 31, 900 Rockville Pike, Bethesda, Md. 20014.

National Kidney Foundation, 315 Park Ave., South, New York, N.Y. 10022.

National Multiple Sclerosis Society, 257 Park Ave., South, New York, N.Y. 10010.

National Parkinson Foundation, Inc., 135 E. 44th St., New York, N.Y. 10017.

National Tuberculosis and Respiratory Disease Association, 101 2nd St., N. E., Washington, D. C. 20002.

Muscular Dystrophy Association of America, 810 7th Ave., New York, N. Y. 10019.

Myasthenia Gravis Foundation, Inc., 230 Park Ave., New York, N. Y. 10017.

United Ostomy Association, 1111 Wilshire Blvd., Los Angeles, Calif. 90017.

*The addresses to these organizations and their policies concerning the sending of materials are subject to change without notice.

## STUDENT INVOLVEMENT
### Investigations
Find out the average costs of a complete medical examination including the recommended laboratory work from the

local medical association. Compare with cost estimates received from individual doctors in your community.

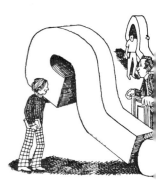

Determine what services the health department provides in screening for chronic and degenerative disease. Are the T.B. unit or other screening units placed for optimum use in community spots? What new screening programs exist for allergies, genetic diseases, or hypertension?

List the heart disease, cancer, or tumor diagnostic clinics in your community, the services they provide, and the cost.

Survey the local public schools to determine the health instruction program relating to chronic and degenerative diseases. Are they adequate?

Check with the health service in your college about examinations they give to prevent or screen for chronic disease.

Start a personal medical history listing familial disease, name and date of past illnesses, findings from last medical examination including types of laboratory examination, and normal temperature, pulse, and blood pressure.

What chronic disorders are caused by venereal diseases? Determine percentage of patients permanently hospitalized because of conditions resulting from syphilis.

How do chronic diseases affect insurance and hospitalization premium costs?

## Action

Volunteer to serve as a patient aide, recreation or music leader in a nearby convalescent home.

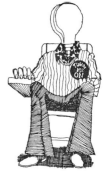

Visit a local rescue squad to see special equipment they may have for first aid care for cardiac patients.

Interview a diabetic student to learn if and how this student may be required to limit his activities and diet. How does he cope with the emotional problems of adjustment?

Visit a "Breathmobile" of the T.B. Association. Take the test, if advisable, and / or interview the medical personnel available on the value of this service.

Volunteer to help a family that has a child affected with a birth defect or other serious health problem. Contact local chapters of voluntary health agencies.

Volunteer to help feed children in a nearby children's home or hospital. It takes a sizeable staff to care for children who cannot feed themselves. Stay around to play with the kids and be a big sister or brother.

## BASIC SOURCE MATERIALS

"Alerting the Public to Heart Attack Signs," *Medical World News*, 14: 18-19, March 9, 1973.

Ardmore, Jane, "Cancer Doesn't Fight Fair," *Family Health*, 8:30-33, 58, September, 1976.

Benke, Paul J., "Screening Newborn Infants for Disease," *Perspectives in Biology and Medicine*, 19:118-23, Autumn 1975.

Berk, Harry, "Diagnosis: Emphysema," *Family Health*, 8:48-49, 74, October, 1976.

"Breaking Down the Barriers to Total Cancer Nursing," *RN*, 41:54-65, April, 1978.

"Cancer in School-Age Children," *Journal of School Health*, special issue, 47:141-84, March, 1977.

Cant, Gilbert, and Toby Cohen, "The Operation Women Never Dreamed Would Be Possible," *Good Housekeeping*, 18:56-68, September, 1975.

Chenoweth, Alice D. "High Blood Pressure: A National Concern,' *Journal of School Health*, 43:307-309, May, 1973.

Elwell, C. C., "The Image of Cancer," *Human Behavior*, 4:41-43, August, 1975.

Fitzpatrick, Genevieve, "Caring for the Patient With Cancer of the Breast," *Nursing Care*, 9:9-15, January, 1976.

Garrison, Webb, "Pain: Your Body's Early-Warning System," *Today's Health*, 47:28-29, 62-66, October, 1969.

Geil, Mark, et al., "The Treatment of Common Cardiac Arrhythmias," *Journal of the American Pharmaceutical Association*, 16:20-29, January, 1976.

Gerson, Elihu, and Anselm Strauss, "Time for Living: Problems in Chronic Illness Care," *Social Policy*, 6:12-18, November/December, 1975.

Gonzalez, Nicholas, "Preventing Cancer," *Family Health*, 8:30-33, 70, 72, 74, May, 1976.

Grant, Alastair, et al., "Questions Behind the Answers: What People Really Want to Know About Cancer," *International Journal of Health Education*, 18:109-118, April/June, 1975.

Heilman, Joan R., "The Epileptic Child—Breaking through the Myths," *Family Health*, 8:26-29, 62, January, 1976.

Herssh, Evan M., et al., "BCG Vaccine and Its Derivatives," *Journal of the American Medical Association*, 235:646-650, February, 1976.

Leff, David, "Epilepsy: Improving the Picture for Patients," *Medical World News*, 16:47-58, October, 1975.

McCleary, Elliott H., "Chronic Pain," *Family Health*, 9:26-29, 56, August, 1977.

Mickel, Hubert S., "Multiple Sclerosis:

A New Hypothesis," *Perspectives in Biology and Medicine,* 18:363-371, Spring, 1975.

Olds, Sally W., "How to Survive a Heart Attack," *Family Health,* 9:34-37, January, 1977.

Rodman, Morton, "Controlling Chronic Liver Disease," *RN,* 39:79-85, January, 1976.

Rosenman, Ray H., and Meyer Friedman, *Type A Behavior and Your Heart,* New York: Alfred A. Knopf, Inc., 1974.

Soika, Cynthia Vaughan, "Gynecologic Cytology," *American Journal of Nursing,* 73:2092-2095, December, 1973.

Walker, Sidney, "Blood Sugar and Emotional Storms: Sugar Doctors Push Hypoglycemia," *Psychology Today,* 9:69-70, 74, July, 1975.

Weisman, Avery D., and J. William Worden, "Psychological Analysis of Cancer Deaths," *Journal of Death and Dying,* OMEGA, 6:61-75, 1975.

## TEST QUESTIONS

### Multiple Choice Items

1. Among a population of 200 million in the United States, about 20,000,000 are affected by: (a) Neurological disorders, (b) Cancer, (c) *Mental and emotional disorders,* (d) Visual impairment, (e) Heart disease.

2. Which of the following conditions or practices has been *least* scientifically related to the rising incidence of cancer? (a) Air pollution, (b) Radiation, (c) Smoking, (d) *Food additives,* (e) Sunlight.

3. A routine at each periodic physical examination should include: (a) Blood pressure, (b) Chest X-ray, (c) Electrocardiogram, (d) Pulmonary function, (e) *All of these.*

4. Multiple sclerosis, a disease that affects persons between 20 and 40 years of age, is a disease of the: (a) Lymphatic system, (b) Joints of the body, (c) *Nervous system,* (d) Blood, (e) Excretory system.

5. Temporary care for acute symptoms of illness include all but one of the following: (a) Never take or give a medicine, (b) Keep the patient in a bed, (c) Relieve pain, (d) Give patient soft foods of a bland nature, (e) *Apply heat packs to affected area.*

6. Which of the following statements regarding hypertension is *least* valid? (a) It is strongly related to the emotions, (b) Overweight individuals have a higher in-

cidence, (c) *It may result in atrophy of the heart itself,* (d) Body chemistry may be related to the cause, (e) There is a strong relationship between cholesterol and hypertension.

7. Arteriosclerosis means: (a) *Hardening of the outer layer of the arteries,* (b) A hardening of brain tissue, (c) Hardening of the veins, (d) A disease of the arteries in which the inner layer of the wall becomes thick and irregular by deposits of fat, (e) A blood clot that forms in a vessel or chamber of the heart.

8. A condition commonly leading to a heart attack is: (a) Collateral circulation, (b) Vigorous exercise, (c) Venous failure, (d) *Coronary arteriosclerosis,* (e) Underweight.

9. A tumor is: (a) The covering of internal and external surfaces of the body, (b) *A mass of new tissue that proliferates wildly,* (c) Chemical agent formed by the body to help destroy cancer, (d) A growth composed mainly of fibrous or fully developed connective tissue, (e) A new growth made up of epithelial cells.

10. In congestive heart failure the victim: (a) Is underweight usually, (b) Has a low level of cholesterol, (c) Is a moderate cigarette smoker, (d) *Has poor respiratory functioning,* (e) Has glandular difficulties.

11. A coronary occlusion is caused by a blood clot in an artery that supplies the: (a) Brain, (b) Lungs, (c) Liver, (d) Kidneys, (e) *Heart.*

12. The two major methods of treating cancer today are: (a) *Surgery and radiation,* (b) Chemotherapy and vaccines, (c) Isotopes and metals, (d) Radiation, (e) None of these.

13. Diabetes is fundamentally a disease of the: (a) Liver (b) Stomach, (c) *Pancreas,* (d) Blood, (e) Kidneys.

14. All but one of the following are symptoms that require immediate attention: (a) *Reflex,* (b) Pain, (c) Sudden weight change, (d) Vision change, (e) Persistent cough.

15. The most common cause of sudden death from heart disease is: (a) Arteriosclerosis, (b) *Coronary occlusion,* (c) Heart murmur, (d) Atherosclerosis, (e) Angina pectoris.

16. Blood pressure is most likely to be increased by: (a) *Emotional stress,* (b) Inactivity, (c) Fatigue, (d) Undernutrition, (e) Fasting.

17. Of the following statements concerning types of cardiovascular disease, which is *least* accurate? (a) Arteriosclerosis is hardening of the arteries, (b) Stroke and apoplexy are terms commonly used to indicate cerebral hemorrhage, (c) Atherosclerosis is strongly related to cholesterol deposits, (d) *Angina pectoris is another name for coronary thrombosis,* (e) Paralysis of a portion of one side of the body frequently results from a stroke.

18. The most readily curable of the following forms of cancer is: (a) Lung, (b) *Skin,* (c) Uterus, (d) Stomach, (e) Breast.

19. The process of colonization or the spreading of cancer cells from an original site to new locations is called: (a) Metabolism, (b) Phagocytosis, (c) *Metastasis,* (c) Antisepsis, (e) Zoonosis.

20. Which of the following is *least* true concerning arteriosclerosis? It: (a) *Is an inevitable manifestation of aging,* (b) May lead to stroke or apoplexy if located in the brain, (c) Is frequently referred to as hardening of the arteries, (d) Appears to be accelerated by high blood pressure, (e) Is substantially more common in the male than the female.

## Matching Items

| | |
|---|---|
| 1. Arteriosclerosis (h) | a. Form of arthritis |
| 2. Pulmonary fibrosis (e) | b. Stroke |
| 3. Gout (a) | c. Cholesterol |
| 4. Emphysema (j) | d. Tumor |
| 5. Apoplexy (b) | e. Shortness of breath |
| 6. Atherosclerosis (c) | f. Wasting of muscle tissue |
| 7. Sphygmomanometer (i) | |
| 8. Neoplasm (d) | g. Hay fever |
| 9. Allergic rhinitis (g) | h. Hardening of the arteries |
| 10. Muscular Dystrophy (f) | i. Blood pressure |
| | j. Damaged lung sacs |

## Essay Items

1. Indicate and briefly describe some of the main causes of disability in the United States.

2. A periodic health examination is important in the early detection of certain chronic and degenerative diseases. Itemize some of the procedures or observations by the physician during the clinical phase of a good health examination. How much does a complete physical exam cost?

3. Symptoms of illness can develop at any time. What are some of the more common signs that disease may be present?

4. Select any two of the following chronic ailments. Briefly describe something of their nature, symptoms, and treatment.

   Allergies, Cerebral Palsy, Emphysema, Gout, Multiple Sclerosis, Parkinson's Disease

5. There are seven danger signals of cancer that have been widely acknowledged as important to know. List five of these signs of possible cancer.

# INFECTIOUS DISEASES

*Part Two* ☙ *Chapter* 17

---

## BEHAVIORAL OBJECTIVES

The Student

- takes the necessary hygienic measures to prevent the spread of pathogenic microorganisms

- obtains recommended immunizations and chemo-prophylaxis against communicable diseases

- identifies the nature of some of the more common communicable diseases

- recognizes that the control of communicable disease requires constant surveillance and vigilance

- prevents the spread of venereal disease by use of self-imposed prevention measures

- supports community health programs that prevent and control communicable diseases

# SUPPLEMENTARY TEACHING AIDS

*Gift of a Lifetime,* color, 27 min. This film shows extensive research, testing and final breakthrough with a successful vaccine for measles. It includes field testing scenes ranging from the Philippines to Jamaica to illustrate the necessary measures in studying the epidemiology and control of a contagious disease. Modern Talking Pictures, 1200 Stout St., Denver, Co. 80204.

*One Way to Better Cities,* color, 29 min. Decayed cities all across the United States present a satire of "America-The Beautiful." Inner cities become jungles for the few remaining residents and easy prey for criminals and land speculators. Tax reform as an alternative to blight is presented in the case example of Smithfield, Michigan.

*Right From The Start,* color, 22½ min. Intended as a motivational film, it depicts individual cases of ignorance of basic immunization needs of children and procrastination. A discussion guide is available: $10.00 rental, Public Affairs Committee, Inc., 22 East 38th Street, New York, N. Y. 10016.

*VD-The Plague of Love,* color, 20 min. This film is based on a spontaneous rap session with college-age young people. Moderated by a nationally known physician, emphasis is on prevention of the number two communicable disease. Association-Sterling Films, 866 Third Avenue, New York, N. Y. 10022.

Sample cartoon posters illustrating the do's and don'ts of sanitary food service. Write to: William Pugsley, Sanitarian, University of Missouri, Student Health Service, Columbia, Mo. 65201.

Various films available on venereal disease from local or state health departments.

Transparency Originals (See Part 3 of Handbook)

## ORGANIZATIONS THAT HAVE MATERIALS *

American Academy of Pediatrics, 1801 Hissman Ave., Evanston, Ill. 60204.

American Lung Association, 1740 Broadway, New York, N. Y. 10019.

American Medical Association, Bureau of Health Education, 535 N. Dearborn St., Chicago, Ill. 60610.

American Public Health Association, 1015 18th St., New York, N. Y. 10019.

Childrens Bureau, U.S. Department of Health, Education, and Welfare, 330 Independence Ave., S. W., Washington, D. C. 20201.

Metropolitan Life Insurance, School Health Bureau, 1 Madison Ave., New York, N. Y. 10010.

National Institute of Allergy and Infectious Diseases, Office of Information, Bethesda, Md. 20014.

National Tuberculosis and Respiratory Disease Association, 101 2nd St., N. E., Washington, D. C. 20002.

Public Inquiries, Center for Disease Control, Atlanta, Ga. 30333.

*The addresses to these organizations and their policies concerning the sending of materials are subject to change without notice.*

## STUDENT INVOLVEMENT

### Investigations

During a week's time, check on how many times you wash your hands before eating.

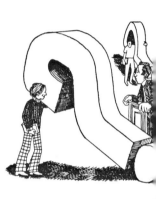

Survey the freshman class to find out what percent are immunized against smallpox, tetanus, polio, mumps, measles. Compare this group with a similar sample of senior students. What might be the reasons underlying your findings?

Inverview a sanitarian to find out how water is purified in your community.

Compare the morbidity and mortality statistics of your community with those of the state and nation.

Check the venereal disease laws in your state regarding treatment without parental consent for minors.

Interview a public health nurse to find out about problems she has with the control of impetigo, pink eye, ringworm, pinworms, and pediculosis in her area.

Check with the health officer about your community's program for venereal disease control. Is the public well informed about the services available?

Investigate the periodic outbreaks of polio in Texas. What might be some causes? Is this phenomena preventable?

What infections are most common in hippie communes? Why? Are they preventable?

*Infectious Diseases*

# Action

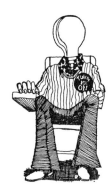

Volunteer to help the local Health Department or March of Dimes with rubella vaccination programs.

Visit a "Free Clinic." Interview doctors or nurses for information on infectious diseases among their patients.

Survey the older people in your community. Ask and record their interpretation of what it was like in the days when cholera, polio, smallpox, diphtheria, T.B. and other diseases struck large numbers of people.

Check on your own immunization record. Are you really protected? If not, make the necessary appointments for innoculations.

## BASIC SOURCE MATERIALS

Barnes, Asa, "Infectious Mononucleosis," *Nursing Digest,* IV, 51-52, January / February, 1976.

Beneson, Abram S., *Control of Communicable Diseases in Man,* New York: American Public Health Association, 1970.

Brenner, Patricia, ed., "Managing the Infectious Pneumonias," *Patient Care,* 9:122-67, December, 1975.

Byron, John Francis, "Current Concepts in Immunization," *American Journal of Nursing,* 73:646-649, 1973.

"Can a Baby's Cold Trigger Crib Death?" *Medical World News,* 17:19-20, February, 1976.

Carper, Jean, "The Case of the Yellow Killer," *(Hepatitis), Today's Health,* 48:53-55, 67-68, September, 1970.

"Child Immunizing Lag Causes Alarm," *Medical World News,* 15:49, August 9, 1974.

Cranston, Lynda, "Communicable Diseases and Immunizations," *The Canadian Nurse,* 72:34-40, January, 1976.

Edelson, Edward, "The Disease Detectives," *Family Health,* 7:27-62, May, 1975.

Fox, John P., Carrie Hall, Lila Elvebach, *Epidemiology: Man and Disease,* New York: Macmillan Co., 1970.

Genell Subak-Sharpe, "The Venereal Disease of the New Morality," *Today's Health,* 53:42, March, 1975.

Leggins, Mary, ed., "Epidemiology: A Mixed Bag of Challenges," *Patient Care,* 10:137-140, January, 1976.

Pariser, Harry and Harry Wise, "Gonorrhea Epidemiology—Is It Worthwhile?" *American Journal of Public Health,* 62:713-14, May, 1972.

Pitman, Naomi, "Measles and Measles," *Life & Health,* 91:30-31, March, 1976.

"Prophylaxis for Rabies With Less Pain, Greater Effect?" *Medical*

*World News,* 14:90e-90h, August, 10, 1973.

Springett, V. H., "Tuberculosis," *Community Health,* 7:66-69, October, 1975.

*Teacher's Manual, A Curriculum Guide on Venereal Disease,* The Commonwealth of Massachusetts, Department of Public Health, Division of Communicable Diseases, 1968.

Thomson, Daniel, "The Ebb and Flow of Infection," *Journal of American Medical Association,* 235:269-272, January, 1976.

"Unvaccinated Kids," *Time,* 106:48, September 8, 1975.

"Vaccines: An Update," *FDA Consumer,* 24-29, December, 1973/ January, 1974.

Van Parijs, Luk, "The Role of Health Education In The Control of Sexually Transmitted Diseases," *International Journal of Health Education,* 18:1-7, July / September, 1975.

"Watch Out for Food Poisoning," *Changing Times,* 29:36-38, August, 1975.

Weaver, J. D., "Is Immunization Necessary? Don't Take A Chance," *Science Digest,* 73:40-43, June, 1973.

Wittle, John, "Recent Advances in Public Health Immunization," *American Journal of Public Health,* 64:939-944.

## TEST QUESTIONS

### Multiple Choice Items

1. The spread of tuberculosis in the United States is intimately related to: (a) Heredity, (b) Climate, (c) *Socioeconomic conditions,* (d) Occupation, (e) Age.

2. The initial sign or symptoms indicating the first stage of syphilis: (a) A small copper colored rash, (b) Nodule-like tissue formed on parts of the body, (c) Pink or white patch-like sores in the mouth,, (d) *A non-painful sore or chancre,* (e) A high temperature.

3. The portal or entry, or the way pathogens most usually enter the body is: (a) Through the respiratory system, (b) Undetectable for many germs, (c) *The same system by which they leave the body,* (d) Through the skin, (e) By food or drink.

4. A positive skin test of Mantoux test shows that a person has: (a) Active tuberculosis, (b) Arrested tuberculosis, (c) *Tuberculosis infection,* (d) Absence of tuberculosis germs, (e) Tuberculosis of the lung.

5. Protection against infection, immunity, which is attained through the body's own reactions to an antigen is called: (a) Natural immunity, (b) *Active immunity*, (c) Passive immunity, (d) Species immunity, (e) Herd immunity.

6. The blood test required by law premaritally and prenatally in most states is to diagnose and prevent: (a) Granuloma inguinale, (b) *Syphilis*, (c) Gonorrhea, (d) Tuberculosis, (e) Chancroid.

7. The study of how disease spreads is known as: (a) Protozoology, (b) Symptomatology, (c) Bacteriology, (d) *Epidemiology*, (e) Parisitology.

8. Infectious mononucleosis is a disease primarily of the: (a) Digestive system, (b) Circulatory system, (c) Nervous system, (d) Reproductive system, (e) *Glandular system.*

9. The causative agents of childhood diseases are most often: (a) Protozoans, (b) *Viruses*, (c) Rickettsiae, (d) Bacilli, (e) None of these.

10. All of the following immunizations for children are recommended except: (a) Diphtheria, (b) *Chickenpox*, (c) Whooping cough, (d) Tetanus, (e) Smallpox.

11. Presently there is no vaccine available for innoculation against: (a) Polio, (b) Measles, (c) Smallpox, (d) Typhoid, (e) *Meningitis.*

12. The essence of tuberculosis control from the public health viewpoint is: (a) *Early-case finding*, (b) Provision of tuberculosis hospitals or isolation wards in general hospitals, (c) Development of drug therapy, (d) Development of chest surgery, (e) Application of BCG immunization to large segments of the population.

13. Which of the following diseases are most likely to be transmitted in drinking water? (a) Malaria and influenza, (b) Scarlet fever and tuberculosis, (c) *Cholera and typhoid fever*, (d) Smallpox and typhus, (e) Yellow fever and leprosy.

14. Infectious mononucleosis is best treated by: (a) *Nothing specific except rest*, (b) Penicillin, (c) Sulfa drugs, (d) Streptomycin, (e) Arsenic Compounds.

15. An individual who is protected against the attack of a specific pathogenic organism is said to be: (a) Resistant, (b) Susceptible, (c) Allergic, (d) *Immune,* (e) Robust.

16. The common cold, pneumonia, influenza, and tuberculosis are all examples of: (a) Viral infections, (b) Chronic infections, (c) Bacterial infections, (d) *Respiratory infections,* (e) Gastrointestinal diseases.

17. Trichinosis is transmitted through: (a) Beef, (b) Lamb, (c) *Pork,* (d) Fish, (e) Fowl.

18. Chemotherapy is: (a) *The use of chemicals to treat disease,* (b) Finding ways in which chemistry can develop new medicines, (c) An ancient form of treatment now scorned by doctors, (d) The application of foreign substances to the skin to draw out the poison, (e) The speciality of graduate training in pharmacy.

19. Of all forms of venereal disease, the most common in terms of incidence is: (a) *Gonorrhea,* (b) Lymphogranuloma, (c) Chancroid, (d) Granuloma inguinale, (e) Syphilis.

20. Antibiotics are effective against: (a) worm infestations (b) viral infection (c) *bacterial and rickettsial infections* (d) bacilli only

## Matching Items

1. Strength of the symptoms of a disease (c)
2. Viral infection (b)
3. Found in warm blooded animals (g)
4. Disease producing organism (b)
5. Isolation (h)
6. Third party spread of disease (j)
7. Contaminated meat (i)
8. Bacterial infection (f)
9. Life that lives off another plant or animal (a)
10. Smallest known parasite (d)

a. Parasite
b. Pathogen
c. Virulence
d. Virus
e. Hepatitis
f. Cholera
g. Rabies
h. Quarantine
i. Salmonellosis
j. Vector
k. None of these

## Essay Items

1. Describe the progress man has made in controlling communicable diseases. Could a science fiction type of world wide epidemic ever happen in the future?

2. List the difference between active and passive immunity.

3. What usually are the effects of advanced cases of syphilis and why is it so hard to treat?

4. List ways diseases are spread and give examples of each.

5. Itemize recommended immunizations for children.

## Discussion Items Concerning Venereal Disease

Various questions arise when we attempt to teach about venereal disease. One of the prime considerations is the question, What do we expect in terms of behavior of the individual as a result of venereal disease education?

*Part I*

*Of the following behavior objectives, select those expectations for individual behavior that are realistic and DISCUSS in relation to the total health behavior of the individual.*

1. Each person will consciously avoid infection by avoiding sexual contacts outside of marriage.

2. Each person will inform himself about venereal disease and if exposed to possible infection, make a positive effort to insure that he is not infected by seeking specific examination for venereal disease by a physician.

3. Each person, if found to be infected, will seek medical treatment, will avoid exposing others to his infection and will make a positive effort to assist in obtaining treatment for those persons from whom he may have contracted the disease and those to whom he may have transmitted it.

4. Each person, if found to be infected, will refrain from sexual relations with others during the infectious stage of the disease.

5. Each person will take positive action to have the disease treated realizing that he is responsible for his own health and his alone.

*Part II*

*Some of the following statements present realistic attitudes that will be prerequisites to the desired behavior in regard to venereal disease. Select those that are realistic. EXPLAIN the validity of the attitude and those factors resulting in the particular attitude.*

1. Each person believes that along with plague, polio, typhoid, smallpox and other diseases, syphilis and gonorrhea are serious and intolerable diseases. They should be regarded objectively, and every citizen should be willing to do what he can to help eradicate them.

2. Syphilis and gonorrhea are only threats to the promiscuous and are of no real concern to the average person except as a general public health problem.

3. Venereal diseases are the result of low moral standards or the sexual revolution and although the person should receive adequate medical care, social censure should be taken against the individual affected.

# SAFETY AND ACCIDENT PREVENTION

*Part Two  Chapter 18*

---

**BEHAVIORAL OBJECTIVES**

The Student

- identifies practices that are potential causes of accidents

- uses behavior that minimizes the chance of having an accident

- recognizes how low levels of emotional and physical well-being predispose to unsafe behavior

- is skillful in the application of first aid of emergency care

# SUPPLEMENTARY TEACHING AIDS

*Before the Emergency*, color, 28 min. This film tells of inadequate care and treatment given by well-meaning, but unprepared persons, and contains information on emergency care and transportation of sick and injured. Modern Talking Pictures, 2323 New Hyde Park Road, New Hyde Park, N.Y. 11040.

*By Nature's Rule*, color, 27 min. This film explains the natural hazards for the unknowing hiker, hunter, or back-packer. As city-bred youth pursue the pleasures of the great outdoors, disaster may strike — sudden storms, wildlife, or rugged terrain. Basic first aid and prevention are explained. Association-Sterling Films, 866 Third Avenue, New York, N. Y. 10022.

*Child Safety Is No Accident*, color, 13 min. Accidents are a leading cause of death in children. This film emphasizes accident prevention and basic first aid if an accident should occur. Major topics covered are burn hazards, poison prevention, auto safety, animal safety, and first aid. Modern Talking Pictures, 3 East 54th Street, New York, N. Y. 10022.

*It Could Happen to You (Rape)*, 27 min. Basic precautionary measures are explained. Medical, police and community counseling services are explained to help the rape victim. Film Library N.R.A., 43 W. 61st Street, New York, N. Y. 10023.

*Snowmobile Safety Savvy*, color, 15 min. The snowmobile is rapidly becoming one of America's most popular winter transportation and recreation vehicles. Viewers can learn the proper way to operate a snowmobile, thus eliminating needless accidents and injuries. Film is done in animated cartoon style and is narrated. Modern Talking Pictures, 3 East 54th Street, New York, N. Y. 10022.

Contact local American Red Cross Chapter for latest films on safety education.

Transparency Originals (See Part 3 of Handbook.)

## ORGANIZATIONS THAT HAVE MATERIALS *

American Automobile Association, Engineering and Safety Department, 1712 G. St., N. W. Washington, D. C. 20016.

American Insurance Association, Engineering and Safety Service, 85 John St., New York, N. Y. 10038.

American National Red Cross, Office of Publications, 17th and D Streets, N.W., Washington, D. C. 20006.

Association of Casualty and Surety Companies, Accident Prevention Department, 60 John St., New York, N. Y. 10038.

Institute of Makers of Explosives, 420 Lexington Ave., New York, N. Y. 10017.

Instructional Materials Laboratories, Inc., Johnson and Johnson, 200 Madison Ave., New York, N. Y. 10016.

Insurance Institute for Highway Safety, 600 New Hampshire Ave., N. W., Washington, D. C. 20036.

Kemper Insurance, Advertising and Public Relations Department, 110 10th Ave., Fulton, Ill. 61252.

Office of Civil Defense, Secretary of the Army, The Pentagon, Washington, D. C. 20310.

The Institute for Safer Living, American Mutual Liability Insurance Company, Wakefield, Mass. 01880.

U.S. Consumer Product and Safety Commission, Bureau of Information and Education, Washington, D. C. 20207.

U.S. Department of Transportation, National Highway Traffic Safety Administration, Washington, D. C. 20590.

*The addresses of these organizations and their policies concerning the sending of materials are subject to change without notice.*

## STUDENT INVOLVEMENT

### Investigations·

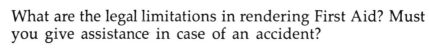

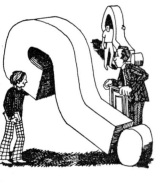

What are the legal limitations in rendering First Aid? Must you give assistance in case of an accident?

Is there a "Good Samaritan" Law in your state? Exactly what does it say?

What is the current First Aid treatment for burns, poisoning, shock and other common emergencies?

What emergency care facilities are available in your home community? Are they adequate?

How much medical treatment or First Aid treatment may

a minor receive without parental consent? Are there exceptions to this?

List the poor driving habits that contribute to driving accidents.

What are the requirements for obtaining a driver's license in your state? How might these be improved? What requirements apply to the handicapped, the elderly?

How does the use of alcohol relate to accidents?

How does the use of marijuana relate to accidents?

## Action

Conduct a survey on campus to find the number of accidents students have had in the past year. What was the seriousness of the injury? What number are related to daily commuting to campus?

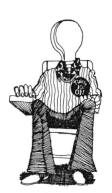

Enroll for a First Aid or Medical Self Help course.

Check your home or dormitory for potential safety hazards. Correct where possible.

Test your reactions while driving. Record distance required to stop at various speeds. The State or local police may have testing instruments that you may use.

Safety check your car.

Install safety belts in your car if you have not yet done so.

Enroll in a defensive driving course.

Visit a junk car lot. Note damage to various autos, type of injury corresponding to passengers.

Conduct a survey to determine effects and value of required driving safety courses for moving vehicle violators.

Survey firearms accidents in your community, county, state. List most common accidents and possible means of prevention. Cite case histories.

Take action to have authorities correct safety hazards in

your neighborhood. Examples: needed traffic lights, street lighting, officer at school crossings, change in speed limits, etc.

Survey available emergency services in your area. Rate. Follow up by sending rate to all services surveyed, local Medical Society, hospitals, and local newspapers.

## BASIC SOURCE MATERIALS

"Auto Safety—Separating the Facts from the Fiction," *Family Health*, 8:36-38, 64, September, 1976.

Bille, Constance, "Winning the Race Against Death," *Family Health*, 7:30-34, 67, 68, August, 1975.

Block, J. R., "Attention Failure: A Test That Tells Who Is Accident-Prone," *Psychology Today*, 9:84-85, June, 1975.

Brooks, Patricia, "Pretty Poison," *Family Health*, 9:29-32, July, 1977.

"Child Abuse Prompts Plan for State Legislative Action," *Intellect*, 101:283-85, February, 1974.

Cleckner, Robert M., "A Long Look At Bicycle Safety," *Journal of Traffic Safety Education*, 23:12-14, October, 1975.

"Community Programs—An Aid to Abused Children," *Intellect*, 102:402-404, April, 1974.

de Roulf, Patty, "Six Driving Nightmares," *Ms.*, 4:88-89, August, 1975.

De Young, Henry, "Homicide" (Children's Division), *Human Behavior*, 5:16-21, February, 1976.

Ellis, Lee, "A Review of Research on Efforts to Promote Occupational Safety," *Journal of Safety Research*, 7:180-89, December, 1975.

Graves, Susan B., "School Sports: How Safe Are They?" *Family Health*, 8:30-33, 60, 62, March, 1976.

"Hard Times for Kids Too," *Time*, Vol. 105:88, March 17, 1975.

Horn, P., "Child-Battering Parent: Sick but Slick," *Psychology Today*, 8:32r, December, 1974.

Howard, Jane, "What Every Woman Should Know About Traveling Alone," *Today's Health*, 52:38-41, 69-70, August, 1974.

Huntley, Henry C., "Emergency Health Services for the Nation," Public Health Reports, 85:517-522, June, 1970.

Kastenbaum, Robert and Laura Briscoe, "The Street Corner: A Laboratory in the Study of Life-Threatening Behavior," *Journal of Death and Dying: OMEGA*, 6:33-34, 1975.

"Medical-Care-on-Wheels will Aid Hospitals and Patients," *Modern Hospital*, 114:78-80, May, 1970.

Naor, Ellen and Raymond Nashold, "Teenage Driver Fatalities Following Reduction in the Legal Drinking Age," *Journal of Safety Research*, 7:74-79, June, 1975.

Nichols, Beverly, "The Abused Wife Problem," *Social Casework*, 57:27-32, January, 1976.

O'Rourke, Thomas W., "The Case for Positive Safety Education," *School Health Review*, 4:35-36, July/August, 1973.

Robertson, Leon, "Safety Belt Use in Automobiles With Starter-

Interlock and Buzzer Light Reminder Systems," *American Journal of Public Health,* 65:1319-1325, December, 1975.

Sadler, Laurie C., "Motorcycling: A Hazardous Two-Wheel Ride," *Today's Health,* 57:28-29, 50, July / August, 1975.

Schoria, Thomas, "Evaluation of Guidelines for Safe Exposure to Continuous Noise of Moderate and High Intensity," *Perceptual and Motor Skills,* 44:307-321, February, 1977.

Shilling, R., "The Place of Occupational Health In the Community," *Occupational Health,* 27:422-425, October, 1975.

Smith, R.C., "New Ways to Help Battering Parents," *Today's Health,* Vol. 51 No. 1 576-580, January, 1973.

Snow, Donald L., "Standard Needs In Controlling Radiation Exposure of the Public," *American Journal of*

*Public Health,* 60:243-49, February, 1970.

"The Abused Child," *Today's Education,* Vol. 63 No. 1 pp. 40-43, January / February, 1974.

"The All-American Blood-Soaked Family," *Human Behavior,* 5:34, 35, February, 1976.

Tofany, Vincent L., Factors Contributing to the Reduction of Motor Vehicle Fatalities in 1974," *Journal of Safety Research,* 7:100-103, September, 1975.

Wingert, W.A., "Changing Trends and Opportunities in Pediatric Emergency Care," *Medical Times,* 98:146-54, May, 1970.

Weisinger, Mort, "Caution: Play It Safe," *Family Health,* 9:44-45, 47, June, 1977.

Williams, Gurney, "Burn Centers— The New Miracle Workers," *Family Health,* 9:48-52, July, 1977.

## TEST QUESTIONS

### Multiple Choice Items

1. The major cause of accidents is: (a) Faulty equipment, (b) Lack of environmental engineering, (c) Insufficient legal regulations, (d) *Poor judgment by the individual of the environment,* (e) Disregard of laws.

2. In recreational activities, the greatest number of deaths occurs while: (a) Hunting, (b) Hiking, (c) *Swimming,* (d) Participation in contact athletics, (e) Any sport that uses metal equipment.

3. The most reliable method of administering artificial respiration is: (a) Back pressure arm lift, (b) Jack-knife, (c) Intermittent abdominal pressure, (d) *Mouth to mouth resuscitation,* (e) Silvester methods.

4. All of the following are recommended precautions to prevent poisoning except: (a) *Wash medicine bottle carefully before reusing,* (b) Don't store medicines with other products, (c) Read labels out loud before taking

a medicine, (d) Keep household chemicals out of the reach of small children, (e) Use only recommended dosages.

5. All of these statements are *false* except: (a) Bullets require a gun to explode, (b) More accidents occur at home than at work, (c) *More fatal accidents occur on the highway than at work or at home*, (d) It is impossible for a person with cramps to swim, (e) Running stream water is safe to drink.

6. Safety experts agree that over what percent of all accidents can be avoided: (a) 50 percent, (b) 60 percent, (c) 70 percent, (d) 80 percent, (e) *85 percent.*

7. The leading fatal accident location for the college student is the: (a) *Highway,* (b) Home, (c) Playfield or gymnasium, (d) Swimming pool, beach or pond, (e) Place of summer employment.

8. It is now recognized that control of traffic accidents rests primarily with: (a) Highway engineers, (b) Car designers and manufacturers, (c) Legislation and enforcement personnel, (d) Teachers of driver education and training programs, (e) *Individual drivers.*

9. The chief causative factor of automobile accidents is: (a) Traffic flow, (b) *Human aspect,* (c) Road design, (d) Laws, (e) Vehicle design.

10. The total economic loss from accidents is many millions of dollars yearly, but more significant is the staggering toll in human life. The number of people who die each year in accidents is approximately: (a) 50,000, (b) 100,000, (c) *150,000,* (d) 200,000, (e) 500,000.

11. All of the following ailments are particularly dangerous for driving except: (a) *Age itself,* (b) High degree of nearsightedness, (c) Night blindness, (d) Glaucoma, (e) Tunnel vision.

12. All of the following are basic rules of water safety, important to help prevent drownings, except: (a) Never swim alone, (b) Inspect the area before diving, (c) Don't swim when overheated or tired, (d) Carry life preservers when boating in deep water, (e) *Swim away from an overturned boat.*

13. The primary problem in recreation safety is: (a) Guns, (b) Fishing, (c) *Drowning,* (d) Outdoor life, (e) Mountain climbing.

14. Of the people who lose their lives in home accidents each year, by far the largest percent of them die as the result of: (a) *Burns and falls,* (b) Inhalation of poison gases, (c) Firearms and electrocution, (d) Suffocation, (e) Falling objects.

15. According to surveys, over one-third of traffic accidents involve: (a) Faulty mechanical conditions of the car, (b) Unfavorable weather conditions, (c) Bad road conditions, (d) *Drinking drivers or pedestrians,* (e) Faulty lights or brakes.

16. The most common substances involved in home childhood poisonings are: (a) *Aspirin, sleeping pills, birth control pills,* (b) Cosmetics, (c) Petroleum products, (d) Pesticides, insecticides, lye, (e) Detergents, lye, acids.

17. When there is severe bleeding, it is usually best to: (a) Apply a tourniquet instantly, (b) Take the person to a doctor, (c) Apply a loose sterile dressing, (d) Immobilize the part that is bleeding, (d) *Apply direct pressure with hand with a clean cloth immediately.*

18. The emotional conflict that seems to occur most frequently among the accident prone is: (a) Remorse and self-accusation, (b) *Aggressiveness and hostility,* (c) Fearfulness and worry, (d) Resentment against authority, (e) Anxiety and guilt.

19. Studies have shown that the universal use of automobile safety belts or seat belts would: (a) Significantly reduce the number of accidents, (b) *Reduce the number of serious and fatal injuries appreciably,* (c) Probably save about 100 lives a year in the United States, (d) Be of little value to the driver behind the steering wheel, (e) Have about the same safety value as padded dashboards.

20. Some drugs, both prescription and nonprescription, may affect one's driving ability by causing: (a) *Drowsiness, visual problems, decreased coordination and alertness,* (b) Drowsiness and decreased alertness, (c) Drowsiness

and hallucinations, (d) No undesirable effects on driving, (e) Optical illusions.

## Matching Items

1. Major cause of traffic accidents (c)
2. Depressed body activities (f)
3. IPPB (g)
4. Attitudes and emotions (e)
5. Reduction in physical capabilities (i)
6. Common cause of childhood accidents (h)
7. Leading cause of death (a)
8. Leading cause of death in 1 to 24 year olds (e)
9. Most often affected by home fires (d)
10. Highest accident rates (b)

a. Heart disease
b. 15 to 24 year olds
c. Fatigue
d. Very young and old
e. Accidents
f. Shock
g. Resuscitation
h. Poisoning
i. Alcohol

## Essay Items

1. Clearly describe the essential procedures involved in giving mouth-to-mouth resuscitation and C.P.R. (cardiopulmonary resuscitation). Indicate some of the things not to do in addition to those steps that should be followed.

2. Carelessness is a well-known cause of accidents. List other prominent causes of accidents and briefly discuss their relationship to the problem. What is meant by "accident proneness"?

3. There are several emergencies or conditions that require immediate first aid. Identify two of these and indicate the first aid procedures that should be followed in each case.

4. Discuss the statements, "Accidents don't just happen —they are caused." Provide some concrete examples to support your thinking.

5. Define what is meant by shock and indicate common symptoms or signs of the condition. What procedures should be followed in first aid care for shock?

6. How can women protect themselves against sexual assault?

# COMMUNITY HEALTH IN ECOLOGICAL PERSPECTIVE

*Part Two & Chapter 19*

## BEHAVIORAL OBJECTIVES

The Student

- recognizes the interrelationships between man and his environment

- identifies community health problems and needs and efforts to help solve them

- analyzes the nature of environmental pollutants

- evaluates how pollutants upset ecological balances

- takes personal responsibility for reducing deleterious effects of pollution

- participates in community activities to reduce levels of pollutants and to help solve other problems

- utilizes community health resources

# SUPPLEMENTARY TEACHING AIDS

*Energy Vs. Ecology . . . The Great Debate,* color, 27½ min. Can we utilize coal, the most abundant source of energy in this country, without disrupting our environment? This film illustrates how land that has been mined can be restored to usable condition. Modern Talking Pictures, 3 East 54th Street, New York, N. Y. 10022.

*Environmental Education—A Beginning,* color, 28 min. Find out what is happening throughout the U.S. in the area of environmental education. Many successful projects are now in progress and perhaps you can learn ways of involving the students at your school. Modern Talking Pictures, 3 East 54th Street, New York, N. Y. 10022.

*The Foresters,* color, 26 min. From the alligator swamps of Georgia to the forests of Oregon, Americans were asked, "What will happen to our forests?" This film recorded many revealing comments by ordinary citizens, foresters, and professional ecologists. Modern Talking Pictures, 3 East 54th Street, New York, N. Y. 10022.

*Forests are for People,* color, 29 min. An interesting and realistic film involving a college student and his experiences with a forester and his family. The future of America's forest resources is speculated. Modern Talking Pictures, 3 East 54th Street, New York, N. Y. 10022.

*King Zog and the Energy Crunch,* color, 19 min. This commonsense approach to energy conservation at home is presented by a funny little king. The film is not academic, but it is educational and motivating where it counts—in everyday energy conservation practices. Association-Sterling Films, 866 Third Avenue, New York, N. Y. 10022.

*Living with Energy,* color, 26 min. This is a documentary dealing with the events and factors leading to the shortage of energy in our environment. One segment of the film suggests ways each sector of our society might cope with the crisis at hand. Modern Talking Pictures, 3 East 54th Street, New York, N. Y. 10022.

*Oil Spill-Pattern in Pollution,* color, 17 min. This film is one of the Sierra Club's most talked about motion pictures. The effects of the relentless search for energy sources—oil, gas, and coal—are dramatically presented. Association-Sterling Films, 866 Third Avenue, New York, N. Y. 10022.

*The Road to Energy, U.S.A.,* color, 29 min. The responsibility for providing and conserving energy in the U.S. rests in the hands of many organizations and individuals. This film allows the viewer to visit several people whose efforts help supply and save the energy in America today. Narrated by a famous celebrity. Modern Talking Pictures, 3 East 54th Street, New York, N. Y. 10022.

*San Francisco Bay*, color, 28 min. Film presents the increasing need for more land for housing, industry, schools, and civic buildings. Landfill is one means; however, how far can we go in destroying irreplaceable resources? Association-Sterling Films, 6644 Sierra Lane, Dublin, Calif. 94566.

*To Protect a Mighty River*, color, 14 min. This film is a welcome change of pace in a world where pollution is destroying our lakes and rivers daily. It concerns the efforts made by one large corporation to reduce the wastes being emptied into the Mississippi River. Modern Talking Pictures, 3 East 54th Street, New York, N. Y. 10022.

*The Trouble With Trash*, color, 23 min. Reveals the ever-growing waste disposal problems facing America. Topics discussed in this documentary are modern sanitary landfills, special incinerators that reduce air pollution, and various recycling techniques. Modern Talking Pictures, 3 East 54th Street, New York, N. Y. 10022.

*Water*, color, 27 min. Explores both the practical and the esthetic use of water and is done in animation with beautiful photography and original music. Topics explored in detail are water pollution, irrigation, chemistry, hydrolic cycle, and conservation. Scientifically oriented. Modern Talking Pictures, 3 East 54th Street, New York, N. Y. 10022.

*"When the Circuit Breaks" . . . America's Energy Crisis*, color, 29 min. Our energy crisis—why did it happen? What are our alternatives now? Development of domestic resources such as coal, oil, and natural gas can solve some immediate problems. But what must be done in the future? Film explores the past, present, and future of the energy crisis in America. Modern Talking Pictures, 3 East 54th Street, New York, N. Y. 10022.

### Filmstrips

*Crisis of the Environment,"* color, with L.P. record. Printed texts and teaching materials. The New York Times Book and Educational Division, Dept. M., 229 W. 43rd St., New York, N. Y. 10036. Topics:

Man—An Endangered Species, Breaking the Biological Strand, Vanishing Species, Preserve and Protect, The Population Explosion.

*Environmental Pollution: Our World in Crisis,* color, 6 filmstrips. A basic presentation of effects of types of pollution and means of control. (1) Nature of the Crisis, (2) Atmospheric Pollution, (3) Land Pollution, (4) Freshwater Pollution, (5) Marine Pollution, (6) Pollution Control. Cat. No. 70W3000. Wards Natural Science Establishment Inc., P.O. Box 1712, Rochester, N. Y. 14603.

*Pollution Simulation Game—"Ecopolis."* In this lively discussion game students assume roles of town manufacturers or the mayor, and as each round of the game is played they must decide how they will run their business and dispose of their waste products. The object is to (1) stay in the game by not going broke, (2) to improve the pollution situation so that the economy and the town may grow. Kit is complete for four groups of 5-9 students playing simultaneously. S.V. Hudson, Office of Environmental Affairs, Continental Can Co., 633 Third Avenue, New York, N. Y. 10017.

Transparency Originals (See Part 3 of Handbook)

## ORGANIZATIONS THAT HAVE MATERIALS *

Aetna Life and Casualty, Public Relations and Advertising Department, 151 Farmington Ave., Hartford, Conn. 06115.

American Lung Association, 1740 Broadway, New York, N. Y. 10019.

American Public Health Association, 1015 18th St., N. W., Washington, D. C. 20036.

Atomic Energy Commission, P.O. Box 62, Oak Ridge, Tenn. 37830.

Audubon Society, 1130 Fifth Avenue, New York, N. Y. 10028.

Department of the Interior, Fishing and Wildlife Service, C St. between 18th and 19th, N. W., Washington, D. C. 20242.

Environmental Protection Agency, 401 M St., S. W., Washington, D. C. 20024.

Environmental Sciences Institute, 125 South Seventh St., San Jose, Calif. 95114.

ERIC Information Analysis Center for Science and Mathematics Education, 1460 West Lane Ave., Columbus, Ohio 43210 (Address to: Dr. Robert E. Roth, Coordinator for Environmental Education).

Exxon Corporation, 1251 Avenue of the Americas, New York, N. Y. 10020.

Food and Drug Administration, Department of Health, Education and Welfare, Washington, D. C. 20025.

National Industrial Pollution Control Council, U.S. Department of Commerce, 14th St. and Constitution Ave., N. W., Washington, D. C. 20230.

National Recreation and Park Association, 1601 N. Kent St., Arlington, Va. 22209.

Office of Environmental Education, Bureau of School Systems, 400 Maryland Ave., S. W., Washington, D. C. 20202.

Population Crisis Committee, 1835 K Street N. W., Washington, D. C. 20019.

Public Affairs Committee, Inc., 22 East 38th St., New York, N. Y. 10016.

Public Health Service, Department of Health, Education and Welfare, Washington, D. C. 20025.

Sierra Club, 1050 Mills Tower, San Francisco, Calif. 94104.

World Health Organization, 505 Park Ave., New York, N. Y. 10022

*The addresses to these organizations and their policies concerning the sending of materials are subject to change without notice.*

# STUDENT INVOLVEMENT

## Investigations

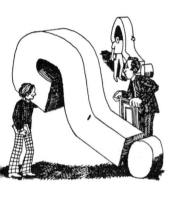

What kinds of public health professionals are represented in the local health departments?

What types of services to individuals are provided by the health department? What are financial eligibility requirements, if any?

Who checks radiation hazards in your community? What academic preparation must they have? Is there an inspection program in industry, in medical laboratories, in physicians' and dentists' offices and in hospitals?

What are the activities for air pollution prevention and control in your community and state?

Survey water resources in your area or state. What steps are being taken to help control pollution?

Conduct an in-depth study of effluent fees. See article "The Economics of Pollution" by Harold Wolozin, *Economic Topic Part III*, Joint Council on Economic Education, 1212 Ave. of Americas, New York, N. Y. 10036. Questions: How will business react to effluent fees? Will politics play a decisive role in administering effluent fees? Would effluent fees be a workable solution?

## Action

Plan a protest or a live campaign in the community for pollution control as needed. Petitions could be circulated to be signed and sent to city, state, and federal officials asking for specific pollution controls needed locally.

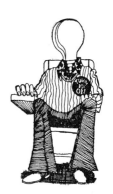

Write anti-pollution radio and T.V. spots and request local stations to tape and broadcast them. Also encourage them to play the record "Pollution" by Tom Lehrer. "The breakfast garbage that you throw into the bay, they drink at lunch in San Jose!"

Clean up an area that needs it. Organize a large student crew with brooms, shovels, etc. Wear work costumes. Request free haul-away service from a local hauler. Contact newspapers, and local radio and T.V. stations ahead of time so that you get good publicity. Have fun doing it. Invite local officials interested in ecology.

Compose songs or original poems on pollution. "Do A Gig" in the student union at lunch time with your songs to alert students to the problems. Hand out literature and litter bags for cars.

Plan a clean-exhaust auto drag race rally. Compute winner based on amount of exhaust, speed, time, distance, etc. Local garages may be able to provide exhaust measuring devices.

Write and distribute an underground newspaper on ecology. Contact *WIN* magazine, 339 Lafayette St., New York, 10012, for ideas.

Survey various neighborhoods, door-to-door, on the topic of community health problems. What problems exist? What, if anything, is being done about the problems? Whose responsibility is it? Compare type of problems in different types of neighborhoods.

Does your state, city, county have certification requirements for homes for the aged? If not, visit several, prepare a suggested inspection form, and personally present it to the proper health officer.

---

## BASIC SOURCE MATERIALS

Alexander, Tom, "What We Know—and Don't Know—About the Ozone Shield," Fortune, 12:184-88, August, 1975.

Berren, James E., "The Abuse of the Urban Aged," *Psychology Today*, 3:37-41, March, 1970.

Carson, Rachel, *Silent Spring*, Greenwich: Fawcett World, 1962.

Cunningham, Wayne, and Virginia Cunningham, "Population Control: A Technological Necessity," *Health Education*, 6:3-4, September/October, 1975.

Deben, Garrett (ed.), *The Environmental Handbook*, Prepared for the Frst National Environmental Teach-in, April 22, 1970, New York: Ballantine, 1970.

Des Lauriers, Lorraine, "Do You Really Need a Yearly Medical Checkup?" *Family Health*, 9:32-34, 51, February, 1977.

"Efficient Solid Waste Disposal: A Civilized Necessity," *Consumer's Research Magazine*, 58:2, 43, September, 1975.

Esposito, John, *Vanishing Air*, New York: Grossman Publishers, 1970.

Fulton, Gere B., "Bioethics and Health Education: Some Issues of the Biological Revolution," *Journal of School Health*, 47:205-11, April, 1977.

Goldsmith, John R., and Erland Jonsson, "Health Effects of Community Noise," *American Journal of Public Health*, 63:782-91, September, 1973.

Gosnell, Mariana, "Ozone—The Trick Is Containing It Where We Need It," *Smithsonian*, 6:48-54, June, 1975.

Graham, Frank, *Since Silent Spring*, Boston: Houghton Mifflin, 1970.

Hahn, Dennis R., and Donald E. Van Farowe, "Misuse and Abuse of Diagnostic X-Ray," *American Journal of Public Health*, 60:250-54, February, 1970.

"Hair Sprays and the Ozone Layer," *Medical World News*, 15:59-61, July, 1975.

Herberger, Roy, "The Ecological Product Buying Motive: A Challenge for Consumer Education," *Journal of Consumer Affairs*, 9:187-95, Winter, 1975.

"High Altitude Data Confirm Ozone Theory," *Science News*, 108:84, August 9, 1975.

"Is Mass Transit Possible?" *Environmental Science and Technology*, 9:816-18, September, 1975.

Kelly, Joseph, "Environmental Education and the Training of Science Teachers," *Science Education*, 59:413-21, July/September, 1975.

Kirkwood, S. S., "In Air Pollution, the Citizen's Voice Counts," *National Tuberculosis and Respiratory Diseases Bulletin*, 56:5-6, June, 1970.

Lehr, Eugene L., "Carbon Monoxide Poisoning: A Preventable Environmental Hazard," *American Journal of Public Health*," 60:289-93, February, 1970.

Lerous, Susan L., "The Driving Hazard You Inhale," *Concepts*, 7:1-4, Fall/Winter, 1974.

"Looking Ahead to the 1970's," *Annual Report 1969*, Washington, D.C.: Resource for the Future, Inc., 1970.

Mennear-Dubas, Susan, "A Startling Report on Hospitals and Doctors," *Family Health*, 9:36-38, August, 1977.

Newman, Ian M., "Some Dilemmas of International Health Education," *Journal of School Health*, 47:94-98, February, 1977.

"Operation Clean Up," *Today's Health*, 54:27-31, February, 1976.

Pines, Wayne, "Polyvinyl Chloride: Why FDA Acted," *FDA Consumer*, 9:5-8, January, 1976.

Prial, Jack, "Rehabilitation through Recreation," *Parks & Recreation*, 11:21-23, 39, February, 1976.

*Ramparts*, "Ecology," special issue, Vol. 8, No. 11, May, 1970.

Robbins, William, *The American Food Scandal*, New York: William Morrow and Company, Inc., 1974.

Roberts, Godrey, "Population Education and Value Analysis," *The Social Studies*, 68:30-32, January/February, 1976.

Russell, Robert D., "Toward a Functional Understanding of Ecology for Health Education," *Journal of School Health*, 39:702-8, December, 1969.

Rutledge, Philip, "The Recession and Urban Population," *Public Welfare*, 33:18-25, Summer, 1975.

Snow, Donald L., "Standard Needs in Controlling Radiation Exposure of the Public," *American Journal of Public Health*, 60:243-49, February, 1970.

Solomon, Stephen, "The FDA: Help or Hindrance," *Family Health*, 10:34-37, 43, March, 1978.

Sultz, H. A., et al., "An Effect of Continued Exposure to Air Pollution on the Incidence of Chronic Allergenic Disease," *American Journal of Public Health*, 60:891-900, May, 1970.

"World Food Supplies and America's Resources: A Review," *Journal of Home Economics*, 67:4-6, November, 1975.

---

# TEST QUESTIONS

## Multiple Choice Items

1. Pollutants that are of particular concern because of their effects on health include: (a) Hydrocarbons, nitrogen oxides, (b) Carbon dioxide, sulfur monoxide, dust and fumes, (c) *Hydrocarbons, nitrogen oxides, dust, fumes, sulfur oxides,* (d) Glycerins, dust and fumes, (e) Carbon monoxide, carbon dioxide, carbon trioxide.

2. If we used the various available techniques to improve water yield and to reclaim water, we might expect: (a) An appreciable increase in supplies, (b) *Only a marginal increase in supplies,* (c) Sufficient supplies to meet the needs of increased technology and population, (d) More water for less expenditure of funds, (e) No appreciable difference.

3. The most widely used method of treating sewage is by:

(a) Screening and sedimentation, (b) Sedimentation, scenting, and adding chemical disinfectants, (c) *Primary treatment, secondary treatment, and chlorination,* (d) Sedimentation, collection, and chlorination, (e) Irrigation.

4. Readily perishable foods should be: (a) Thoroughly cooked before eating, (b) Stored at freezing temperatures, (c) Stored below body temperature, (d) *Stored below 45°F or cooked above 140°F,* (e) Disposed of.

5. Scientists recommend a wide range of new techniques for treating water. Which of the following is *not* a recommendation that has been used: (a) Solvent extraction, (b) *Population redistribution,* (c) Freezing, (d) Electrodialysis, (e) Foaming.

6. Polluted air is linked as a cause of all but: (a) Reduced visibility, (b) Eye irritation, (c) Lung cancer, (d) *Pneumonia,* (e) Emphysema.

7. The most feared and perhaps most important of all the fallout isotopes with respect to radiation is the one called: (a) Carbon-14, (b) Potassium-131, (c) Cesium-137, (d) Calcium-202, (e) *Strontium-90.*

8. By far the major source of radiation to the average person is from: (a) Cosmic rays, (b) Body tissues, (c) Conditions inherent in occupations, (d) Immediate surroundings, (e) *Medical examinations.*

9. Of the general types of substances known to pollute the atmosphere, the one of major concern is: (a) *Chemical,* (b) Radioactive, (c) Meterological, (d) Biological, (e) Rural.

10. Virtually all water supply has its origin in: (a) Lakes, (b) Ponds, (c) Rivers, (d) *Rainfall,* (e) None of these.

11. The primary reason for the marked fall in the underground water level throughout the country is: (a) Increased domestic use, (b) *Urban-suburbanization,* (c) Normal geological change, (d) Abnormal drought, (e) Radioactivity.

12. The greatest danger of water pollution is from: (a) Chemical compounds, (b) *Human wastes,* (c) Animal

wastes, (d) Organic matter of plant life, (e) Salt water intrusion.

13. The science of ecology involves the study of: (a) The interrelationships within the animal kindgim, (b) The interrelationships within the plant kingdom, (c) The interrelationships between the animal and plant kingdom, (d) *The relationships between living things and their surroundings,* (e) The relationships between inert matter and viable matter.

14. All but one of the following is a responsibility of the State Health Departments: (a) Detection and prevention of adulteration of food and drugs, (b) Examination for, and the prevention of, pollution of public water and ice supplies, (c) *Licensing of General Practitioners,* (d) Licensing of hospitals and nursing homes, (e) Preparation and distribution of antitoxins, vaccines and other prevention of communicable diseases.

15. The National Air Sampling Network is designed to provide information on air pollution throughout the country. It is operated by the: (a) *U.S. Public Health Service,* (b) National Safety Council, (c) U.S. Department of Agriculture, (d) Atomic Energy Commission, (e) U.S. Food and Drug Administration.

16. At the state level, which department is usually responsible for air control programs: (a) Building, (b) Fire, (c) *Health,* (d) Public Safety, (e) Education and Welfare.

17. Public health research programs of the Department of Health, Education and Welfare are chiefly centered in: (a) Office of the Surgeon General, (b) *National Institutes of Health,* (c) Bureau of Medical Services, (d) Bureau of State Medical Services, (e) Division of Special Health Services.

18. The World Health Organization maintains its American headquarters in: (a) Canada, (b) United States, (c) *Mexico,* (d) Argentina, (e) Brazil.

19. In the United States, the greatest power in public health matters is vested in (a) Federal government, (b) *States,* (c) Cities, (d) Counties, (e) Courts.

20. Which of the following hidden sources of radiation is

probably the least hazardous: (a) X-rays for medical and dental purposes, (b) Mass chest X-ray programs, (c) Shoe-fitting flouroscope, (d) *Old black and white television sets,* (e) Radium dial watches and clocks.

## Matching Items

1. Radioactive materials (d)
2. Contaminated air (g)
3. Warm air above colder air (h)
4. Food poisoning (c)
5. Radioisotopes (j)
6. Insecticides (i)
7. Motor vehicle exhausts (b)
8. Organisms discharged from humans (e)
9. Pesticide (a)
10. Fuel oil burners (f)

a. Parathion
b. Hydrocarbons
c. Botulism
d. Contaminants
e. Coliforms
f. Sulfur-oxides
g. Smog
h. Inversion
i. Toxic aerosols
j. Tracers
k. None of these

1. United Nations (c)
2. U.S. Department of Health, Education & Welfare (f)
3. Animal disease (g)
4. Chief Officer, Public Health Service (j)
5. Former head of American Heart Association (h)
6. First State Board of Health (b)
7. World Health Organization (i)
8. Poliomyelitis (e)
9. Consolidated fund raising (a)
10. Labor Department (d)

a. Community Chest
b. Massachusetts
c. UNICEF
d. Children's Bureau
e. Jonas Salk
f. Public Health Service
g. Brucellosis
h. Robert Wilkins
i. World Health Assembly
j. Surgeon General
k. New York
l. Louis Pasteur
m. None of these

## Essay Items

1. Indicate three different types of sewage systems that are utilized to help control water pollution.

2. List four specific activities of the federal government to help prevent and control air pollution.

3. Identify some of the specific substances that contribute to the air pollution problem in the United States.

4. List the major functions of the local health department. Are these functions sufficient to meet current needs?

5. List four major sources of radiation in the United States that may be hazardous to health.

6. What is the role of the State Health Department? What is your evaluation of the effectiveness of your State Health Department?

7. Discuss some international controls that might contribute to solutions to pollution problems. What people and / or organizations other than government might initiate interest internationally, and how might they go about achieving their objectives.

8. Why is interest in world health a necessity today?

9. How can schools contribute to heathful living in a community?

10. What role should the voluntary health sector play in the future health of the nation?

11. Describe the structure and activities of the World Health Organization.

# RETROSPECT AND PROSPECT IN HEALTH

*Part Two* ❦ *Chapter 20*

---

## BEHAVIORAL OBJECTIVES

The Student

- analyzes the changes that are occurring in the provisions of health services and the implications for health education of the public

- summarizes the important contributors and contributions to health through the ages

- identifies issues and controversies about providing health services

- believes that the individual can still influence social events

- illustrates some of the discoveries and events that reflect recent progress in health and offer greater hope for the future

# SUPPLEMENTARY TEACHING AIDS

*Automania 2000,* color, 10 min. An imaginative approach to the problem of traffic congestion as it is foreseen at the turn of the century. The film shows a worldwide affluent society that has become one giant traffic jam. For some of us, not too far from reality. Contemporary Films, McGraw-Hill, 828 Custer Ave., Evanston, Ill. 60202.

*The City—A Study in Survival,* color, 28 min. Industrial pollution is a worldwide problem. This film presents practical ways of making a city livable in one of the densest industrial centers of Germany. Urban renewal and environmental conservation projects are discussed. Association-Sterling Films, 866 Third Avenue, New York, N. Y. 10022.

*No Room for Wilderness,* color, 26 min. The rapid disappearance of the world's wilderness areas is cause for alarm. This film shows the impact of technical civilization and the population explosion on the natural ecological cycle. Association-Sterling Films, 866 Third Avenue, New York, N. Y. 10022.

*Health through the Ages,* chart and booklet, Metropolitan Life Insurance Company, One Madison Avenue, New York, N. Y. 10010.

*Great Moments in Medicine,* book and poster series, Parke Davis Company, Detroit, Mich. 48232.

*1985,* 56 min., color, 3 parts for discussion purposes. A fictionalized newscast demonstrating the projected effects of continued destruction of the environment. Order No. MM-101. CCM Films, 860 Third Avenue, New York, N. Y. 10022.

*Sorry No Vacancy,* color, 27 min. Will man be able to increase the food and energy supply as fast as population growth? This film explores alternatives and features short interviews with some of the nation's leading scientists. Malibu Films, Inc., P.O. Box 428, Malibu, Calif. 90265.

Transparency Originals (See Part 3 in Handbook).

## ORGANIZATIONS THAT HAVE MATERIALS *

The American Health Foundation, Inc., 320 East 43rd St., New York, N. Y. 10017.

American Medical Association, Bureau of Health Education, 535 N. Dearborn St., Chicago, Ill. 60610.

American Association for the Advancement of Science, 1515 Massachusetts Ave., N. W., Washington, D. C. 20005.

Association for the Advancement of Health Education, 1201 16th St., N. W., Washington, D. C. 20036.

American School Health Association, 107 Depeyster St., P. O. Box 416, Kent, Ohio 44240.

Consumer Product Safety Commission, 5401 Westbard Ave., Room 100, Washington, D. C. 20207.

Hastings Center, 360 Broadway, Hastings-on-Hudson, N. Y. 10706.

Health Policy Advisory Council, 17 Murray St., New York, N. Y. 10007.

Science Research Associates, Inc., 155 N. Wacker Drive, Chicago, Ill. 60606.

Society for Public Health Education, Inc., 655 Sutter St., San Francisco, Calif. 94102.

National Institute of Child Health and Human Development, Office of Research Reporting, Building 31, Room 2A-34 NIH, Bethesda, Md. 20014.

*The addresses to these organizations and their policies concerning the sending of materials are subject to change without notice.

## STUDENT INVOLVEMENT
### Investigations

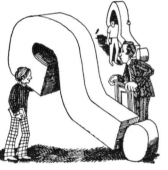

Investigate and report the biography of a prominent modern-day scientist who contributed to the improvement of health.

Although man's well-being has been greatly improved through science, what kinds of problems related to health and safety have in turn been created by science and technology?

What are some of the reasons for the apparent lag between discovery and application of new health findings? How might this gap between knowledge and actual use be shortened or eliminated?

What were some unwanted side effects of oxygen administration to premature babies? Why do so many preemie babies now wear strong corrective lenses?

What are new foods or food substances being developed? Will the potential supply meet the demand?

What might be some contributing factors to explain the apparent increase in birth defects? Radiation, drugs, pollution?

Develop a paper highlighting health conditions that existed

in ancient Egypt, classical Greece, the Renaissance, Colonial America, or another period of history.

Explore the responsibility that the individual will have for his own health in the future. Possible self-diagnosis with machines, and computer drug prescriptions?

## Action

Prepare an exhibit on the topic of the city of the year 2050, one lifetime from now.

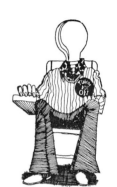

Write and present a short dramatization of "A Day in the Life of Joe Doe, Year 2000."

Visit a comprehensive, modern diagnostic center that uses computers and other modern equipment to perform a complete physical examination or for intensive care units.

As a class, develop a "time line" or wall chart indicating some of the contributors and contributions to health, medicine, and science through the ages.

Call the president of the student body of a medical school. Make arrangements to meet with a group of medical students to learn of their commitment, their views on medical practice, the quality of their training, etc.

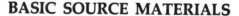

## BASIC SOURCE MATERIALS

Belson, Abby A., "Predictive Medicine," *Family Health*, 7:30-33, January, 1975.

Blum, Albert A., "Automation, Education and Unemployment: Some Safety Valves," *Phi Delta Kappan*, 51:554-57, June, 1970

Brennan, Andrew, "Employment Prospects of Future Health Educators," *The American College Health Association*, 24:66-67, December, 1975.

Chernow, Ron, "Colonies in Space May Turn Out to Be Nice Places to Live," *Smithsonian*, 6:62-68, February, 1976.

Dolfman, Michael L., "Toward Operational Definitions of Health," *Journal of School Health*, 44:206-9, April, 1974.

Engel, G. G., "Grief and Grieving," *American Journal of Nursing*, 64:93-98, September, 1974.

Fiilop, Tamas, Ed., "Manpower for National Health: Needs, Planning, Implementation," *Impact of Science on Society*, 25:213-24, July/September, 1975.

Hurster, Madeline, "Critical Issues in Health Education," *Journal of School Health*, 47:42, January, 1977.

Hutchins, Vince L., "New Policies in School Health," *Journal of School Health*, 47:428-30, September, 1977.

Insel, Paul, and Rudolf H. Moos, *Health and the Social Environment*, Lexington, Mass. 02173, D. C. Heath and Company, 1974.

"Is Health Planning Too Vital to Be Left up to MD's?" *Medical World News*, 11:17-18, July 31, 1970.

Jackson, Edgar N., *Telling a Child about Death*, New York: Channel Press, 1965.

Jones, Syl, "How Would You Deal with Disaster?" *Modern Medicine*, 43:51-60, December, 1975.

Kahn, Joel S., Rosalyn M. Cain, and Sydney P. Galloway, "Planning in Poverty Areas," *Journal of American Pharmaceutical Association*, 10:466-68, August, 1970.

Kennedy, Edward M., "Preventive Medicine—What It Can Mean for You," *Family Health*, 8:40-42, 62, 64, January, 1976.

Lampe, David, "Physicians and Physicists—Far-Out Medicine," *Family Health*, 9:48-50, September, 1977.

Martino, Joseph, "Forecasting Technological Breakthroughs," *The Futurist*, 4:101-2, June, 1970.

Mayur, Rashmi, "The Coming Crises in Third World Cities," *The Futurist*, 9:108-74, August, 1975.

McClendon, E. J., "America's Health in Two Centuries," 47:271-73, May, 1977.

Means, Richard K., *Historical Perspectives in School Health*, Thorofare, N.J.: Charles B. Slack, Inc., 1975.

Merrill, Jeffrey, "Planning for New Health Humanpower," *Social Policy*, 6:36-43, November/December, 1975.

Miller, C., "Societal Change and Public Health: A Rediscovery," *American Journal of Public Health*, 66:54-66, January, 1976.

Orleans, Myron, and Florence Welfeson, "The Future of the Family," *The Futurist*, 4:48-49, April, 1970.

Russell, O. R., *Freedom to Die*, New York: Human Sciences Press, 1975.

Schaller, Warren E., "School Health at the Crossroads: An Introduction," *Journal of School Health*, 47:393-94, September, 1977.

Scheinberg, Labe, "Pulling the Plug—A Matter of Life," *Family Health*, 8:47-48, 56, March, 1976.

"Special Feature: Aging—A New Opportunity for Health Education," *Health Education*, 6:2-18, July/August, 1975.

"State Laws May Ease Malpractice Ills," *Patient Care*, 10:18-34, January, 1976.

Stevens, Robert, and Rosemary Stevens, *Welfare Medicine in America*, New York: Free Press, 1974.

"The Test that Could Save Your Life," *Family Health*, 8:44-57, December, 1976.

Tisdell, C., "The Theory of Optimal City Sizes," *Urban Studies*, 12:61-70, 1975.

Volkan, Vamik D., "Move on Re-Grief Therapy," *Journal of Thanatology*, 3:77-91, 1975.

"When Should Life Be Prolonged?" *Science News*, 108:48, October 4, 1975.

## TEST QUESTIONS

### Multiple Choice Items

1. In infant mortality rates, the United States rates behind most other Western Countries and Russia as: (a) Third,

(b) *Fifteenth,* (c) Twentieth, (d) Twenty-fifth, (e) Fiftieth.

2. The poor rates that the United States maintains in infant mortality and heart-artery disease can be accounted for by: (a) Outdated hospital equipment and practices, (b) Poor quality care in teaching hospitals, (c) Shortage of medical personnel, (d) *Poor health conditions of certain groups of people,* (e) Inadequate health insurance plans.

3. The "Satellite System" of medical care means: (a) *A ring of community health centers and rural medical out-post stations,* (b) Regional medical centers, (c) Heart-cancer-stroke diagnostic centers under the administration of the Public Health Service, (d) Proposed future medical centers for astronauts, (e) Medicare.

4. At the present time there are approximately how many million people in the United States? (a) One Hundred, (b) *Two hundred,* (c) Three hundred, (d) Four hundred, (e) Five hundred.

5. The chief polluter of the air in the United States is: (a) *The automobile,* (b) Home incineration, (c) The mining industry, (d) Agriculture, (e) The road paving industry.

6. The "green revolution" refers to: (a) *High-yield wheat and rice grains,* (b) Air pollution, (c) The berets in Viet Nam, (d) Water pollution, (e) New systems of medical care.

7. L-dopa is a drug that has proved effective as a chemical treatment for the disease: (a) Leprosy, (b) Tuberculosis, (c) *Parkinsonism,* (d) Malaria, (e) Cancer.

8. Three and a half billion people represents the number of the world: (a) *Population,* (b) Malnourished, (c) Maternal deaths, (d) Polluted cities, (e) Infant deaths.

9. Rubella is another name for: (a) Whooping cough, (b) Influenza, (c) *German measles,* (d) Pneumonia, (e) Mumps.

10. The National Health Test conducted on television in 1966 disclosed that approximately what percent of

those taking the test believed that it is possible to catch venereal disease from toilet seats? (a) 10 percent, (b) 25 percent, (c) *40 percent*, (d) 50 percent.

11. One paradox in the health field is that: (a) The increase in life expectancy has reduced illness, (b) *The decline in mortality rate has not reduced illness*, (c) Greater longevity has decreased morbidity rates, (d) Fatality rate is due to greater longevity, (e) Medicine has not decreased the morbidity rate.

12. The largest number of individuals rejected by the Army are turned down because of: (a) *Disease or defects of the bones or limbs*, (b) Flat feet, (c) Diabetes, (d) Eye diseases and defects, (e) Feeblemindedness.

13. Technological changes have produced new public health problems. An example is: (a) Fire hazards, (b) Alcoholism, (c) Mental illness, (d) Increase in diseases, (e) *Radiation*.

14. The National Health Test conducted on television in 1966 disclosed that approximately what percent of those taking the test could not name even three of the danger signals of cancer: (a) 15 percent, (b) 35 percent, (c) 55 percent, (d) *75 percent*, (e) 95 percent.

15. The high cost of medical care has led to an: (a) *Expansion of health insurance*, (b) Increase in medical students, (c) Intense interest and time spent on important patients, (d) Increase in hospital and office facilities, (e) Intense desire to prevent illness.

16. The most vulnerable age groups for disease today are the: (a) Infant and school age child, (b) Adolescent, (c) Adolescent and early adult, (d) Infant and adolescent, (e) *Infant and middle age.*

17. The prevention of illness is becoming more a matter of: (a) Controlling environmental conditions, (b) *Changing the habits and customs of people*, (c) Immunizing the population, (d) Controlling alcoholism and drug addiction, (e) Informing the people by fear.

18. If farmers today used 1940 methods, it would cost approximately how many billion dollars a year to produce

food for the nation: (a) Less than five, (b) *Thirteen*, (c) Twenty, (d) Thirty, (e) Over fifty.

19. The study of population shows that people: (a) Have not been informed of available health facilities, (b) Accept illness and early death as natural, (c) Are finally beginning to cooperate with health officials, (d) *Are beginning to demand health services in their own communities*, (e) Are taking steps to avoid future diseases.

20. Major health problems in the United States have shifted in the past fifty years: (a) From childhood to adolescent disease, (b) From females to males, (c) From the rich to the poor, (d) *From communicable to chronic and degenerative diseases*, (e) From old age diseases to heart disease.

21. The pattern of individual illness today requires: (a) *Prevention, early detection, and rehabilitation measures*, (b) Immunization programs for large numbers of people, (c) Surgery and medical treatment, (d) General public health codes and regulation, (e) Emergency care.

22. The most recent public health and safety crusaders have been: (a) Upton Sinclair, Jessica Mitford, Louis Pasteur, (b) *Rachel Carson, Ralph Nader, Edmund Muskie, Jessica Mitford*, (c) Upton Sinclair, Rachel Carson, Robert Kennedy, Alexander Fleming, (d) Jonas Salk, Mary S. Calderone, John Rock, Allan Guttmacher, (e) Jonas Salk, John Enders, René Dubos.

23. The most spectacular gains in enactment of health legislation today seems to result from the impetus of: (a) Health professionals and agencies, (b) Concerned individuals, (c) Medical schools and teaching hospitals, (d) *Concerned individuals, pressure groups, and aroused public*, (e) Lobbyists in Washington.

24. Project HOPE, the medical ship provided to needy countries for a specific period of time, is sponsored by: (a) United Nations Assembly, (b) United States government, (c) Peace Corps, (d) World Health Organization, (e) *Gifts and donations from private citizens*.

25. The main sources of health information for the general public are usually: (a) *Medical television programs and commercials*, (b) Compulsory Health Education courses at all grade levels in schools, (c) Public health nurses,

(d) The classroom teacher, (e) Medical journals and magazines.

26. A paradox of current spectacular advances in medical science and technology is: (a) It is easier for the physician to practice, (b) *It is more difficult for the physician to practice*, (c) People no longer trust physicians, (d) There is an over supply of medical personnel, (e) There is less demand for medical care.

27. Medical welfare services in many states are now beginning to offer services to: (a) The "indigent" only, (b) *The "respectable poor" as well as to the "indigent poor,"* (c) Anyone employed at the time of need, (d) No one except mothers and children on welfare rolls for at least a year.

28. Which of the following assumptions about the attitude of the poor toward family planning has been found true in various research studies: (a) The poor do not want birth control, (b) The poor will not accept birth control measures even if available, (c) *The poor want and will utilize family planning information and services when made available*, (d) Procreation is the poor man's recreation, (e) The poor want large families.

29. Ranked with other western countries, the U.S. stands: (a) First in life expectancy, (b) *Twelfth in life expectancy*, (c) Twenty-fifth in life expectancy, (d) Fiftieth in life expectancy.

## Matching Items

| | |
|---|---|
| 1. Team medicine (d) | a. Laser beam |
| 2. Stress of modern living (f) | b. Suicide |
| 3. Army rejections (g) | c. Neonate |
| 4. Behavior changes (i) | d. Group practice |
| 5. Newly born (c) | e. Technological changes |
| 6. Shortage of personnel (h) | f. Increase in mental illness |
| 7. Social deviance (b) | |
| 8. New health problems (e) | g. Health problem in United States |
| 9. Public interest in medical matters (j) | h. Inadequate medical care |
| 10. Seals broken blood vessels (a) | i. New methods of health education |
| | j. Increase in health articles |

## Essay Items

1. The advances in medicine have been spectacular in recent years. What are some of the modern medical advances that have improved health?

2. Discuss some of the major changes that have taken place with respect to the nature of disease.

3. The astounding developments in the health-related fields have improved well-being, but likewise, have created new problems. Indicate some of the medical paradoxes or difficulties in relation to advances that have taken place in recent years.

4. Identify and briefly elaborate upon some of the recent changes that have occurred in medical care practices and organization.

5. Public health practice has undergone some transformation during the modern era. What are some of these changes? What implications might be derived from these influences?

6. What age-old philosophical questions must be answered as new developments and medical-technical skills are developed? What might be some guides for arriving at solutions? Who must make some of these decisions—the physician, the patient, the patient's family?

# Part Three

Included in this section is a collection of visual masters, or printed originals, basically of a pictorial nature. These can be used in their present form or be duplicated for individual or small-group study. Or, as is recommended, they can be developed into transparencies for viewing with an overhead projector. Guidelines for developing and using transparencies are given.

# Chapters

*21 Guidelines for Transparencies*

# GUIDELINES FOR TRANSPARENCIES

*Part Three* ৰ্ঠ *Chapter 21*

## ADVANTAGES OF
## TRANSPARENCY USE

Overhead projection of transparencies is one excellent way to enrich and enliven health instruction. It incorporates simplicity and ease of use with optimum effectiveness. Its use in teaching is limited only by the ingenuity and imagination of the instructor.

It is for these and other reasons that the authors have chosen to provide original materials for use with the overhead projector. Other advantages of the approach include the following:

Transparency projection can be used in a completely lighted room and still be clearly seen by all students.

The teacher can face the class at all times, since the overhead projector is placed at the front rather than the rear of the classroom.

Transparencies are widely adaptable and can be used as a chalkboard by writing on them, to reveal point-by-point ideas by simple coverage of portions of the projected material, and to incorporate other techniques.
The projector is light in weight and relatively easy to handle for transportation from class to class.

Transparencies made with a copying machine are permanent teaching aids that can be used many times without erasure or fading.

## MAKING TRANSPARENCIES

The construction of transparencies for overhead projection is a simple process. All that is needed are original drawings or pictures, blank transparencies, and a copying machine. A number of originals are provided in this handbook for the various units of instruction. Others can easily be made by following these steps:

Use a plain sheet of paper and a soft lead pencil.

Draw the desired illustration or use other prepared black line drawings from magazines or newspapers (numerous figures appearing in the professional or popular literature can be used effectively).

Print or type captions for each transparency where desired, using letters of at least one-fourth inch.

Overlay this original with a blank transparency and merely run both through the copying machine. This step is all that is required for the originals included in this handbook.

Color may be added to the transparency by using color adhesive film or felt-tipped pens.

Sequences, successive steps, or multiple operations can be demonstrated by the use of overlay transparencies, each step added to the prior one by merely flipping the overlay into place.

# TRANSPARENCY MASTERS

Health Education (chart)
Health Shopper—Beware
Consumer Health
Interrogatives of Evaluation
Endocrine Definitions
Endocrine Glands
Causes of Tooth Decay
Selecting an Activity
Isometric—Isotonic
Symptoms of Fatigue
Nutrition Nonsense
Prevention of Fatigue
This is What Happens When a
    Fly Lands on Your Food
Frustration by Thwarting
Psychoneurotic Disorders
Psychoses
Misconceptions about Alcohol
Varying Effects of Alcohol
Effects of Alcohol
Dr. Tobias Venner
Factors Causing Variances
    in Tobacco
Recommended Steps to Lower
    One's Intake of Cigarette
    Smoke

Why People Use Drugs
Drug Abuse Problem
Drug Addiction—20th Century
Drug Effects
An Old Persian Tale
The Family Life Cycle
World Record
Hemorrhage
Spasm
Compression
Embolism
Thrombus
Disease Prevention and Control
Immunity
The Disease Process
Why Safety?
Causes of Accidents
Three E's of Accident
    Prevention
Air Pollution
Effects of Air Pollution
Why Air Pollution?
Types of Health Agencies
Leading Causes of Death in the
    United States
Life Expectancy

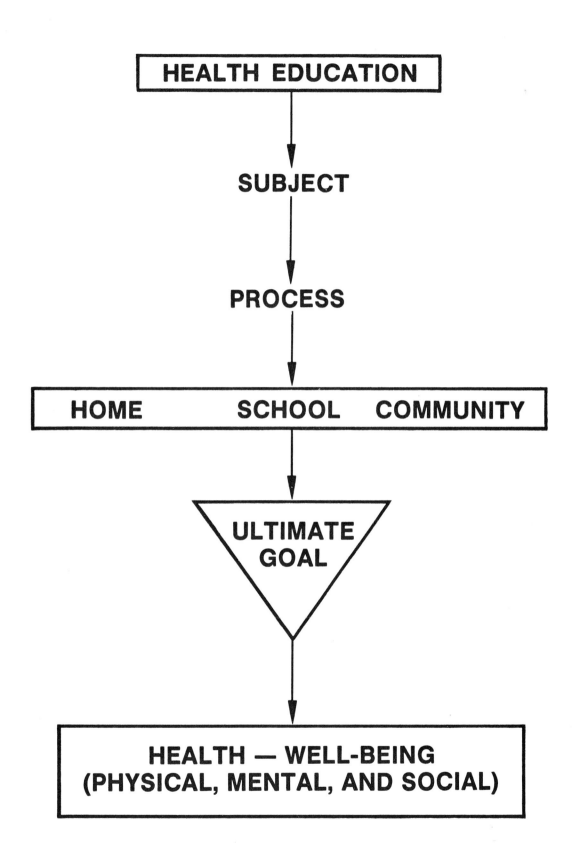

# HEALTH SHOPPER.....

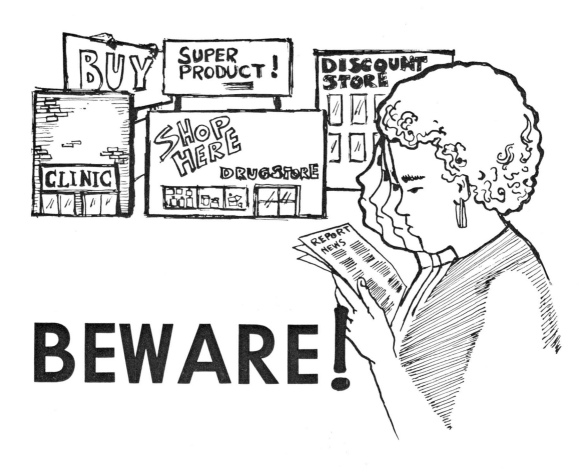

# BEWARE!

# CONSUMER HEALTH

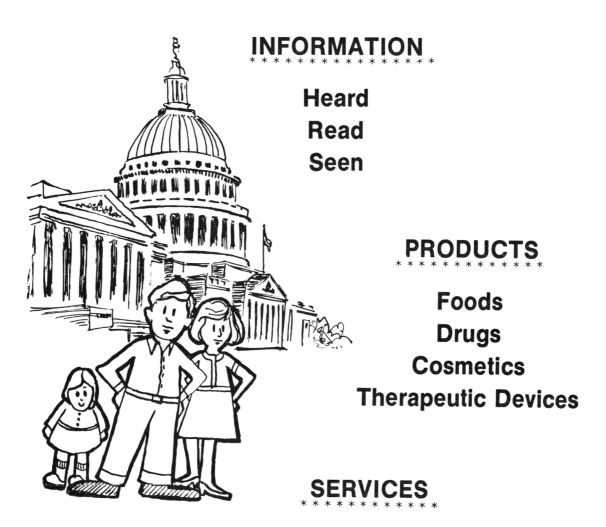

## INFORMATION
* * * * * * * * * * * * *

**Heard**

**Read**

**Seen**

## PRODUCTS
* * * * * * * * * * * *

**Foods**

**Drugs**

**Cosmetics**

**Therapeutic Devices**

## SERVICES
* * * * * * * * * * *

**Quacks and Quackery**

**Health Personnel**

**Hospitals and Clinics**

**Health Insurance**

**Medical Care**

# INTERROGATIVES OF EVALUATION

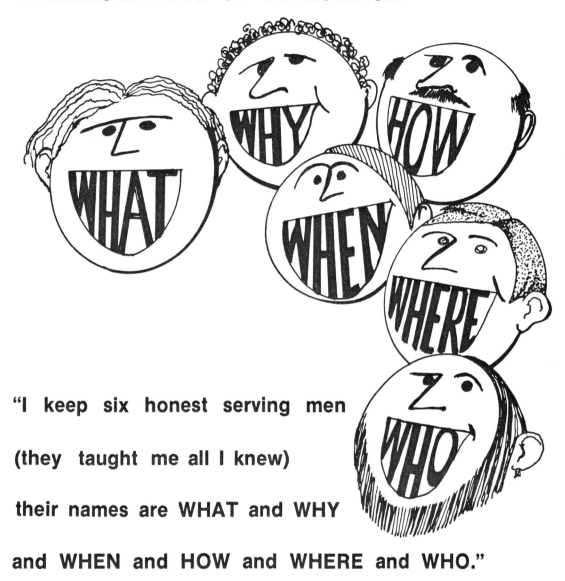

"I keep six honest serving men

(they taught me all I knew)

their names are WHAT and WHY

and WHEN and HOW and WHERE and WHO."

**Rudyard Kipling, <u>Just So Stories</u>**

*ENDOCRINE* — **MEANS "SECRETING IN-TERNALLY"**

*ENDOCRINE GLANDS* —
## GLANDS OF INTERNAL SECRETION "DUCTLESS GLANDS"

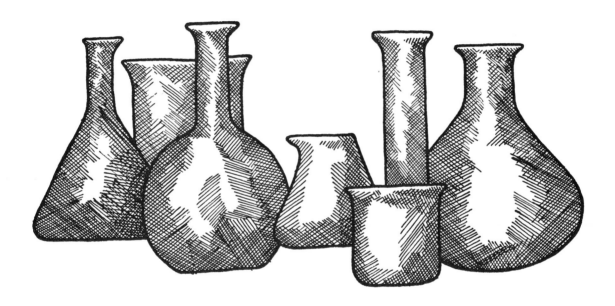

*HORMONES* —
## SECRETIONS OF ENDOCRINE GLANDS SECRETE DIRECTLY INTO THE BLOOD OR LYMPHATIC SYSTEM

# ENDOCRINE GLANDS

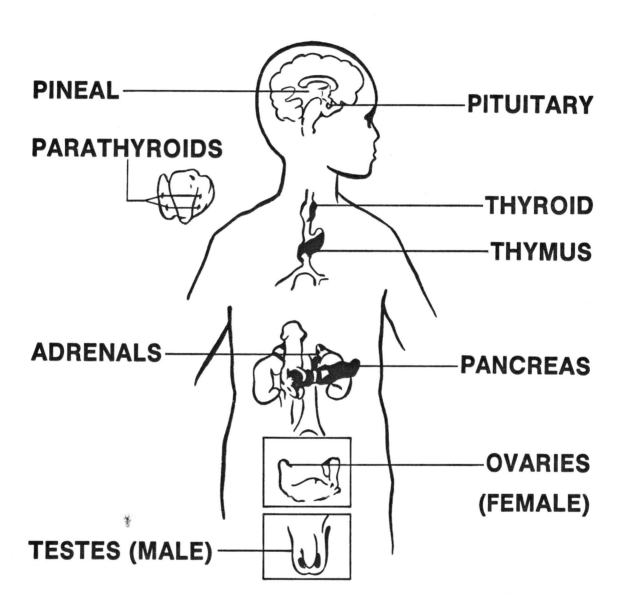

PINEAL

PITUITARY

PARATHYROIDS

THYROID

THYMUS

ADRENALS

PANCREAS

OVARIES
(FEMALE)

TESTES (MALE)

# CAUSES OF TOOTH DECAY

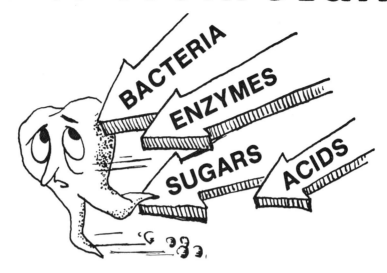

**ENAMEL — SUSCEPTIBILITY TO DECAY
HEREDITARY IMPLICATIONS**

**BACTERIA — PRODUCE ACIDS AND EN-
ZYMES THROUGH ACTION ON SUGARS**

**SUGARS — FERMENTABLE CARBOHYDRATE
CONSUME 10 TIMES THE AMOUNT
OF 100 YEARS AGO**

**ENZYMES — PRODUCED BY BACTERIA**

**ACIDS — PRODUCED BY BACTERIA
VARY IN STRENGTH**

# SELECTING AN ACTIVITY

**PROMOTES STAMINA AND ENDURANCE**

**CAN BE CONVENIENTLY SCHEDULED**

**YEAR-ROUND ACTIVITY**

**ONE CAN AFFORD**

**FUN AND ENJOYABLE**

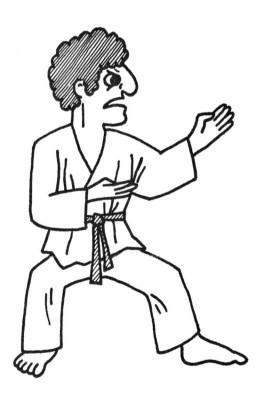

**AVOID OVEREXERTION**

**MINIMIZE RISK OF INJURY**

**WARM-UP PROPERLY**

**TAPER OFF GRADUALLY**

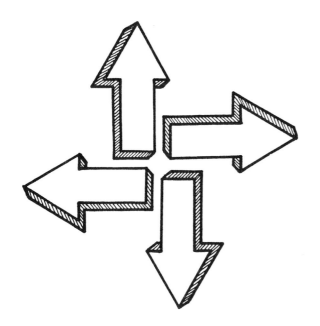

# ISOTONIC

## TRADITIONAL EXERCISE

## INVOLVES MOVEMENT

# ISOMETRIC

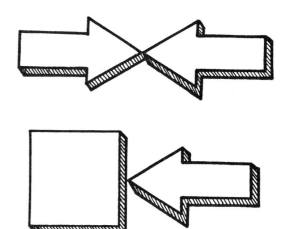

**NO MOVEMENT**

**PERFORMED AGAINST AN IMMOVABLE OBJECT**

# SYMPTOMS OF FATIGUE

LOSS OF WEIGHT

PALENESS

SUSCEPTIBILITY TO INFECTION

LACK OF INTEREST

SHORTNESS OF BREATH

RESTLESSNESS

DESIRE TO BE ALONE

EXHAUSTION

IRRITABILITY

DIFFICULTY IN SLEEPING

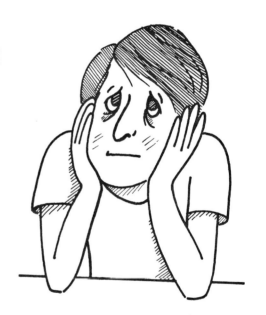

# NUTRITION NONSENSE

**ALUMINUM PANS CAUSE CANCER**

**FRIED FOODS ARE INDIGESTIBLE**

**DARK BREAD IS MORE NUTRITIOUS THAN WHITE BREAD**

**OLEOMARGARINE IS LESS FATTENING THAN BUTTER**

**WATER AT MEALS INTERFERES WITH DIGESTION**

**TOAST IS LESS FATTENING THAN BREAD**

**EGGS, OYSTERS AND OLIVES PROMOTE FERTILITY**

**VITAMIN B CURES HANGOVERS**

# PREVENTION OF FATIGUE

**HIGH LEVEL OF FITNESS**

**SOUND MENTAL HEALTH**

**GOOD ATTITUDES**

**ADEQUATE SLEEP**

**CHANGE OF PACE ACTIVITIES**

**SOUND DIET AND NUTRITION**

**PROPER REST AND RELAXATION**

**GOOD SCHEDULE AND PLANNED
DAILY ROUTINE**

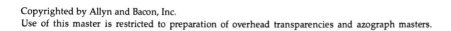

# THIS IS WHAT HAPPENS WHEN A FLY LANDS ON YOUR FOOD

FLIES CAN'T EAT SOLID FOOD, SO TO SOFTEN IT UP THEY VOMIT ON IT.

THEN THEY STAMP THE VOMIT IN UNTIL IT'S A LIQUID, USUALLY STAMPING IN A FEW GERMS FOR GOOD MEASURE.

THEN WHEN IT'S GOOD AND RUNNY, THEY SUCK IT ALL BACK AGAIN, PROBABLY DROPPING SOME EXCREMENT AT THE SAME TIME.

AND THEN, WHEN THEY'VE FINISHED EATING, IT'S YOUR TURN.

# FRUSTRATION BY THWARTING

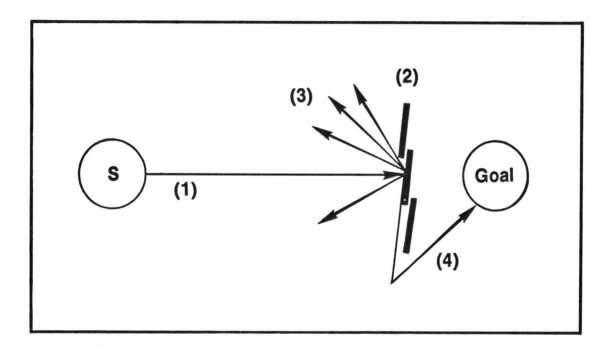

*Frustration by Thwarting.* **An organism (S) is motivated to approach (1) a goal. It encounters a barrier (2), is thwarted and tries various responses (3). One response successfully gets around the barrier. (4).**

# PSYCHONEUROTIC DISORDERS

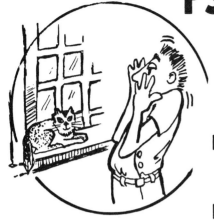

**NEURASTHENIA**

**HYSTERIA**

**ANXIETY NEUROSIS**

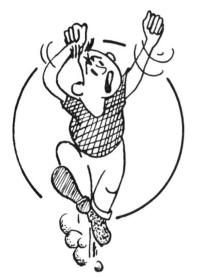

**PHOBIAS**

**OBSESSIONS**

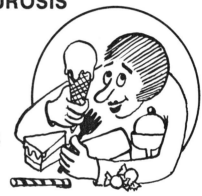

**COMPULSIONS**

**ADJUSTMENT BY AILMENT**

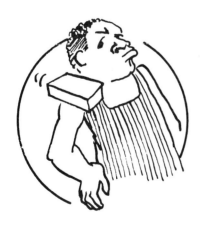

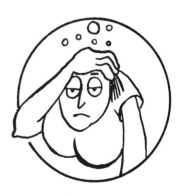

# PSYCHOSES

**SCHIZOPHRENIA**

**MANIC-DEPRESSION**

**INVOLUTIONAL MELANCHOLIA**

**PARESIS**

**TOXIC DELIRIA**

**PSYCHOSES OF OLD AGE**

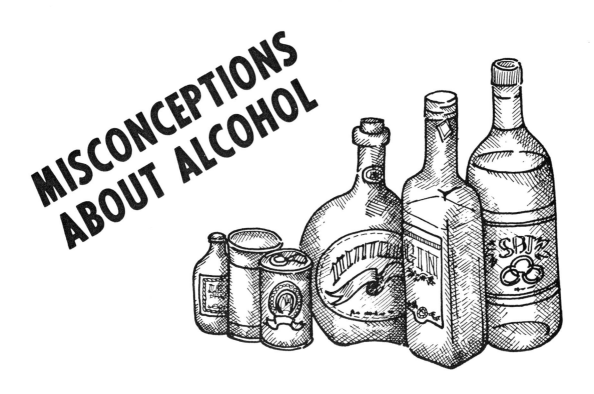

# MISCONCEPTIONS ABOUT ALCOHOL

**ALCOHOL INCREASES THE ABILITY TO THINK**

**A DRINK WILL HELP CURE A COLD**

**ALCOHOL IS A STIMULANT**

**ANYONE WHO REALLY WANTS TO CAN CONTROL HIS DRINKING**

**ALCOHOL HAS NO CALORIC VALUE**

**ALCOHOL SPEEDS REACTION TIME**

# VARYING EFFECTS OF ALCOHOL

TYPE OF BEVERAGE CONSUMED

LENGTH OF DRINKING TIME

SIZE OF THE PERSON

AMOUNT CONSUMED

FOOD EATEN

MENTAL STATE

FATIGUE

OTHER FACTORS

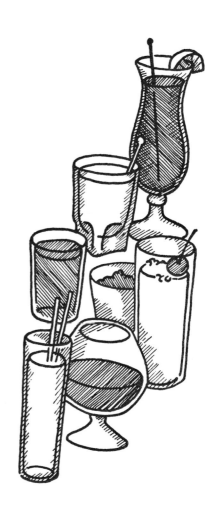

# EFFECTS OF
# ALCOHOL

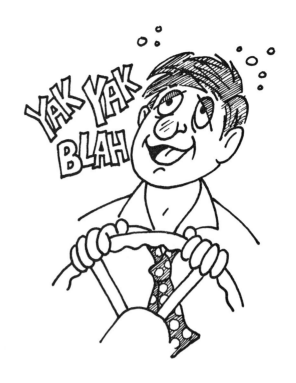

**0.1 - 0.2    EFFECT ON MENTAL SKILLS
TALKATIVE
0.15 IS UNSAFE DRIVER (N.S.C.)**

**0.2 - 0.3    EFFECT ON PHYSICAL SKILLS
IMPAIRED JUDGMENT**

**0.3 - 0.5    EFFECT ON SENSORY PER-
CEPTIONS
BALANCE AND RELATED ACTIVITIES
LOSS OF CONSCIOUSNESS**

**0.5 - 0.7    DEATH**

## DR. TOBIAS VENNER, 1620

"IT DRIETH THE BRAIN, DIMMETH THE SIGHT, VITIATETH THE SMELL, DULLETH AND DEJECTETH BOTH THE APPETITE AND THE STOMACH, DISTURBETH THE HUMORE AND SPIRITS, CORRUPTETH THE BREATH, INDUCETH A TREMBLING OF THE LIMBS, EXSICCATETH THE WINDPIPE, LUNGS AND LIVER, AND SCORCHETH THE HEART."

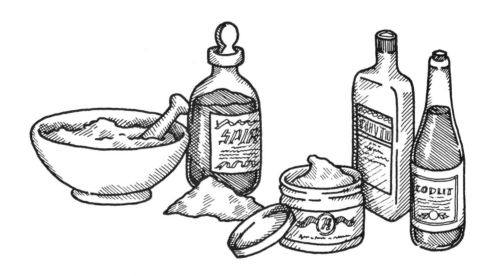

## DR. EVERARD, 1659, London, England

RECOMMENDED THE USE OF TOBACCO LEAVES, EXTRACTS, OINTMENTS, POWDERS AND LOTIONS TO CURE AN ALMOST ENDLESS LIST OF HUMAN ILLS, WHICH INCLUDED HEAD-ACHES, DEAFNESS, TOOTHACHES, COUGHS, STOMACH PAINS, BURNS, WOUNDS, WORMS, AND MAD-DOG BITES.

# FACTORS CAUSING VARIANCES IN TOBACCO

SOIL THE TOBACCO IS GROWN IN

METHODS OF PROCESSING THE LEAF

DRYNESS OF THE TOBACCO

RATE AT WHICH TOBACCO IS SMOKED

HOW THE TOBACCO IS SMOKED

HOW THE CIGARETTE IS PACKED

HOW FAR THE CIGARETTE IS SMOKED TO THE END

# RECOMMENDED STEPS TO LOWER ONE'S INTAKE OF CIGARETTE SMOKE

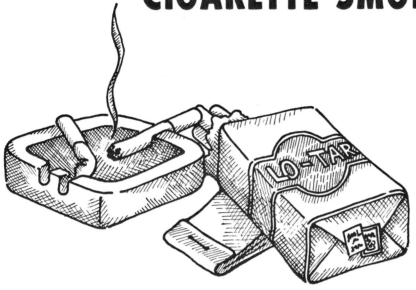

**CHOOSE A CIGARETTE WITH LESS TAR AND NICOTINE**

**DON'T SMOKE THE CIGARETTE ALL THE WAY DOWN**

**TAKE FEWER DRAWS ON EACH CIGARETTE**

**REDUCE YOUR INHALING**

**SMOKE FEWER CIGARETTES PER DAY**

# WHY
# PEOPLE USE DRUGS

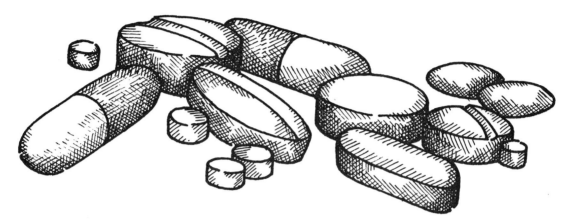

## MEDICAL REASONS (PAIN RELIEF)

## IGNORANCE (LACK OF KNOWLEDGE)

## PERSONALITY DISORDERS (NEUROTIC)

## REBELLION AGAINST AUTHORITY

## GROUP PRESSURE (NEED TO BELONG)

## CURIOSITY (THRILL SEEKING)

## ESCAPE (FROM PROBLEMS, DIFFICULTIES)

M-23

# DRUG ABUSE PROBLEM

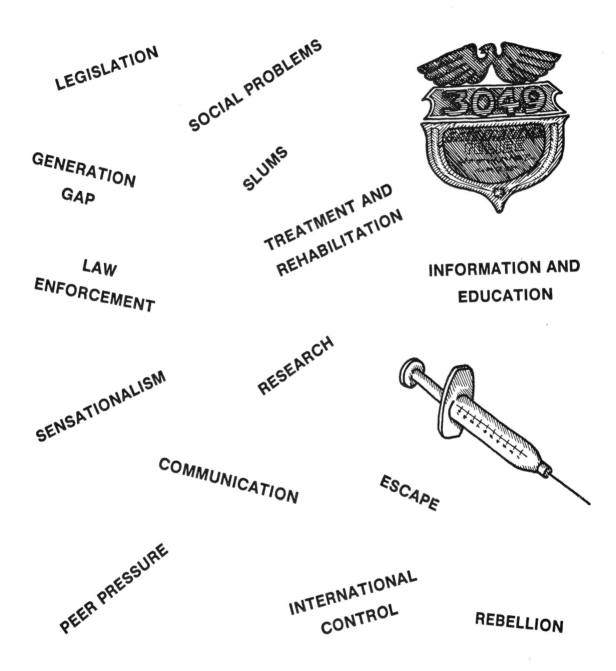

LEGISLATION

SOCIAL PROBLEMS

GENERATION GAP

SLUMS

TREATMENT AND REHABILITATION

LAW ENFORCEMENT

INFORMATION AND EDUCATION

RESEARCH

SENSATIONALISM

COMMUNICATION

ESCAPE

PEER PRESSURE

INTERNATIONAL CONTROL

REBELLION

# NO. REPORTED ADDICTS

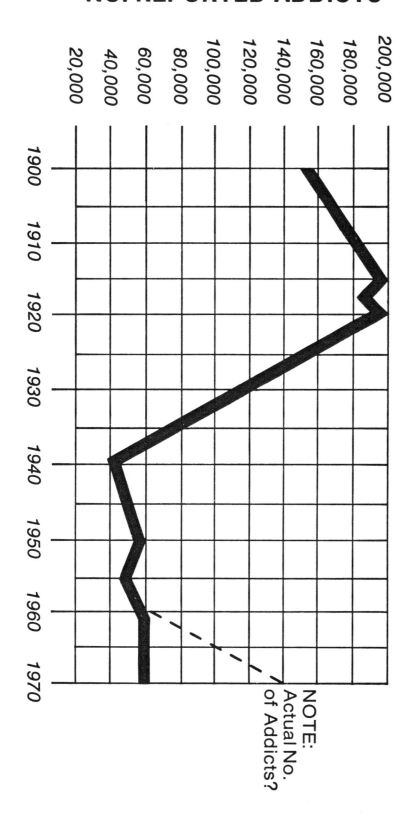

DRUG ADDICTION—20th CENTURY

200,000
180,000
160,000
140,000
120,000
100,000
80,000
60,000
40,000
20,000

1900  1910  1920  1930  1940  1950  1960  1970

NOTE:
Actual No.
of Addicts?

# DRUG EFFECTS

**POOR GENERAL HEALTH STATUS**
**MALNUTRITION**
**INFECTION, BOILS, BLOOD POISONING**
**STERILITY (inability to have children)**

| DISEASES — | MALARIA | PNEUMONIA |
|---|---|---|
| | ULCERS | HEPATITIS |
| | SYPHILIS | TUBERCULOSIS |
| | TETANUS | BRONCHITIS |

**POSSIBILITY OF SUDDEN DEATH**
**DECREASED LIFE EXPECTANCY**

. . . . . . . . . . . . . . . . . . . . . . . .

**CHANGE IN PERSONALITY**
**LOSS OF RESPONSIBILITY**
**CRIMINAL ACTIVITY**
**SCHOOL DROP-OUT, LOSS OF JOB**

# AN OLD PERSIAN TALE, STILL TOLD TODAY IN SOUTHWESTERN ASIA

THREE MEN ARRIVED AT ISPAHAN AT NIGHT. THE GATES OF THE TOWN WERE CLOSED. ONE OF THE MEN WAS AN ALCOHOLIC, ANOTHER AN OPIUM-ADDICT, AND THE THIRD TOOK HASHISH.

THE ALCOHOLIC SAID: "LET US BREAK DOWN THE GATE."

THE OPIUM SMOKER SUGGESTED: "LET US LIE DOWN AND SLEEP UNTIL TO-MORROW."

BUT THE HASHISH-ADDICT SAID: "LET US PASS THROUGH THE KEYHOLE."

WORLD HEALTH Magazine, 13: 24, January-February, 1960.

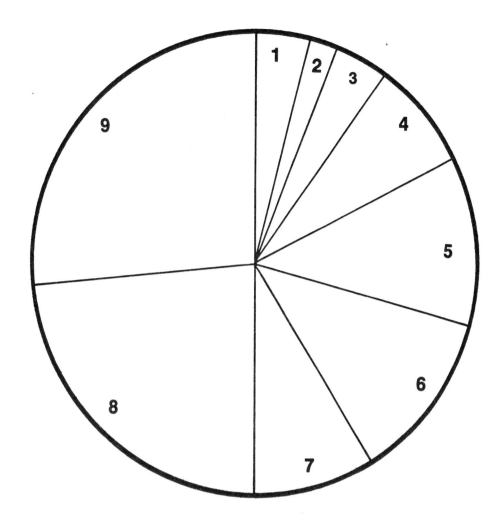

# THE FAMILY LIFE CYCLE

1. **Newly Married Pair**
2. **Expectant Parents**
3. **Parenthood (1st Child)**
4. **The Crowded Years**
5. **The Early School Years**
6. **Adolescent School Years**
7. **The Launching Years**
8. **The Empty Nest**
9. **The Aging Years**

# WORLD RECORD

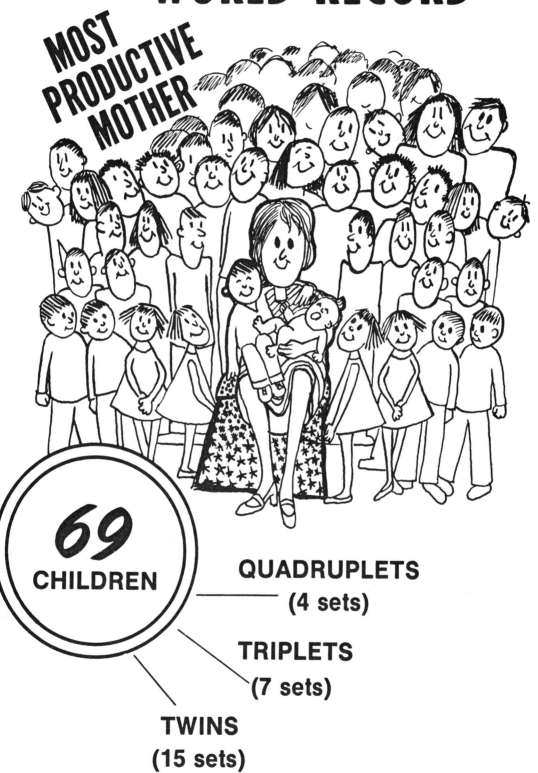

MOST PRODUCTIVE MOTHER

**69 CHILDREN**

QUADRUPLETS (4 sets)

TRIPLETS (7 sets)

TWINS (15 sets)

# HEMORRHAGE
## (BLEEDING)

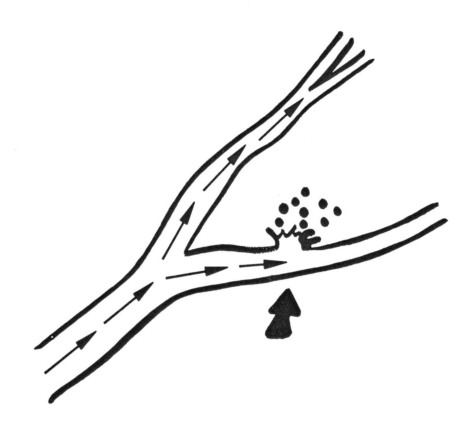

## THE WALL OF AN ARTERY
## MAY BREAK, PERMITTING BLOOD
## TO ESCAPE AND THUS DAMAGE
## SURROUNDING TISSUE

# SPASM

## (Tightening and Closing Down of the Walls of an Artery)

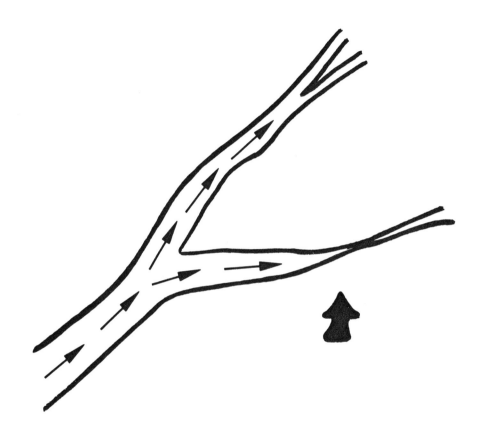

AN ARTERY MAY CONSTRICT
AND THUS REDUCE THE FLOW
OF BLOOD TO AN AREA. IF THE
SPASM IS OF SHORT DURATION THEN
PERMANENT DAMAGE DOES NOT NECES-
SARILY OCCUR.

# COMPRESSION
## (PRESSURE)

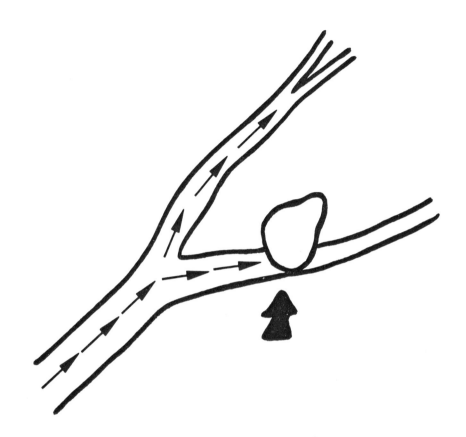

A TUMOR, SWOLLEN TISSUE,
OR LARGE CLOT FROM ANOTHER
VESSEL MAY PRESS UPON A VESSEL
AND STOP ITS NORMAL FLOW OF BLOOD.

# EMBOLISM

## (Blocking of a vessel by a clot floating in the blood stream)

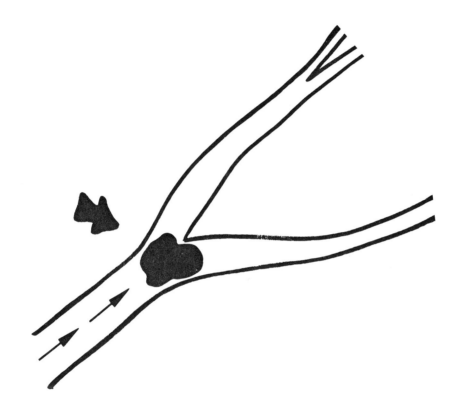

## A CLOT FROM A DISEASED HEART OR, LESS COMMONLY, FROM ELSEWHERE IN THE BODY MAY BE PUMPED TO ANOTHER LOCATION AND STOP UP AN ARTERY.

# THROMBUS

## (CLOT FORMATION)

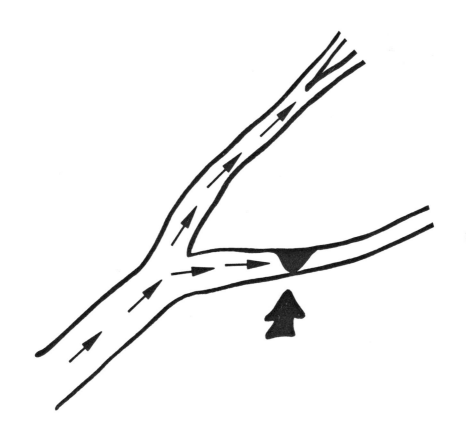

## A CLOT OF BLOOD MAY
## FORM IN AN ARTERY AND
## MAY STOP THE FLOW OF BLOOD
## TO THE PART OF THE BODY
## SUPPLIED BY THE CLOT-PLUGGED ARTERY

# DISEASE PREVENTION AND CONTROL

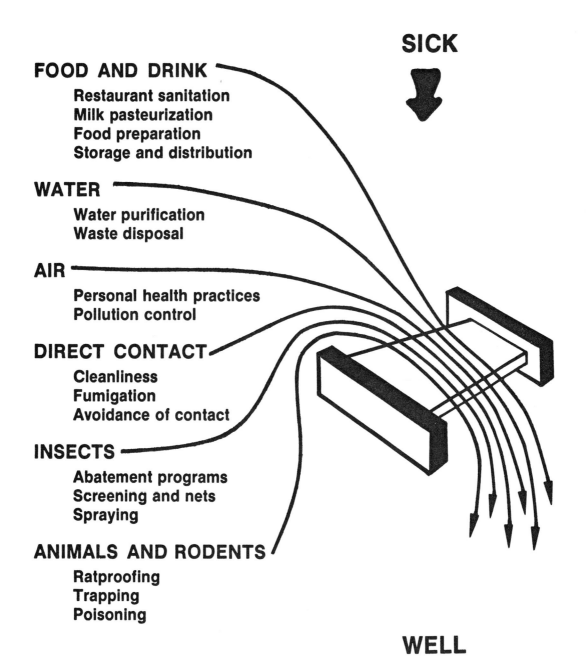

SICK

**FOOD AND DRINK**
- Restaurant sanitation
- Milk pasteurization
- Food preparation
- Storage and distribution

**WATER**
- Water purification
- Waste disposal

**AIR**
- Personal health practices
- Pollution control

**DIRECT CONTACT**
- Cleanliness
- Fumigation
- Avoidance of contact

**INSECTS**
- Abatement programs
- Screening and nets
- Spraying

**ANIMALS AND RODENTS**
- Ratproofing
- Trapping
- Poisoning

WELL

# IMMUNITY

__IMMUNITY__ — THE ABILITY TO RESIST
   A SPECIFIC DISEASE

__SUSCEPTIBILITY__ — PRONENESS TO DISEASE

__RESISTANCE__ — THE GENERAL ABILITY TO
   RESIST DISEASE

IMMUNITY IS BASED UPON THE IDEA
OF FINDING AND THEN INTRODUCING A
SUBSTANCE INTO THE BODY WHICH WILL
REACT OR STIMULATE THE PRODUCTION
OF ANTIBODIES AGAINST A SPECIFIC
DISEASE

# THE DISEASE PROCESS

THE INDIVIDUAL IS CONTINUOUSLY EX-POSED TO PATHOGENS

THEY SOMETIMES GAIN ENTRY TO THE BODY

THE PATHOGEN GROWS AND MULTIPLIES

THE BODY DEFENSES SET UP OBSTACLES TO DESTROY OR WARD OFF THE DISEASE

IF THE ORGANISM WINS, SYMPTOMS DEVELOP

IF THE BODY WINS, DISEASE HAS BEEN AVERTED

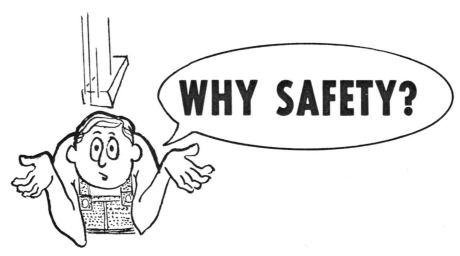

**WHY SAFETY?**

## CHANGING SOCIAL CONDITIONS AND PRACTICES

## SCIENTIFIC AND TECHNOLOGICAL ADVANCES

### NEW IMPLEMENTS AND TOOLS
### HIGH SPEED TRANSPORTATION

## GIANT STRIDES IN INDUSTRIAL DEVELOP-MENT

## INCREASING POPULATION

## GROWTH OF LARGE CITIES AND SUBURBS

## DIFFERING PROBLEMS TODAY

# CAUSES OF ACCIDENTS

CARELESSNESS AND INATTENTION

PHYSICAL DISABILITY AND ILLNESS

DRINKING AND INTOXICATION

FATIGUE

MECHANICAL FAILURE

ENVIRONMENTAL CONDITIONS

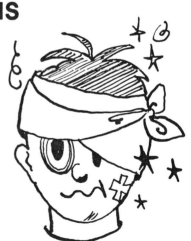

EXCESSIVE SPEED

IGNORANCE

EMOTIONAL INSTABILITY

# THREE E'S OF ACCIDENT PREVENTION

EDUCATION — TO DEVELOP INDIVIDUAL RESPONSIBILITY AS WELL AS SKILLS AND PROPER SAFETY HABITS

ENGINEERING — TO HELP MAKE THE PHYSICAL CONDITIONS AND SURROUNDINGS AS SAFE AS IS HUMANLY POSSIBLE

ENFORCEMENT — OF LAWS GOVERNING SAFE CONDUCT AND OF REGULATIONS DE-SIGNED TO PREVENT ACCIDENTS

# AIR POLLUTION

**SMOG — SMOKE AND FOG (CALIFORNIA)**

**SMAZE — SMOKE AND HAZE (NEW YORK)**

**SMUST — SMOKE AND DUST (TEXAS)**

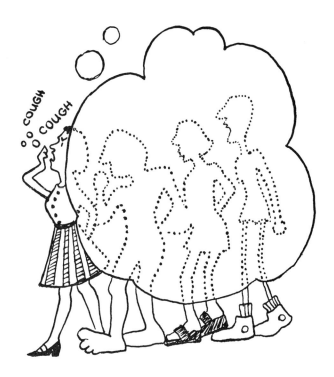

# EFFECTS OF AIR POLLUTION

**INTERFERENCE WITH VISIBILITY**

**SOILING OF CLOTHES AND MATERIALS**

**CROP (PLANT) DAMAGE**

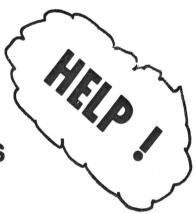

**RESPIRATORY AILMENTS**
  **LUNG CANCER**
  **CHRONIC BRONCHITIS**
  **EMPHYSEMA**

**IRRITABILITY AND EMOTIONAL TOLL**

**NOXIOUS ODORS**

**EYE AND THROAT IRRITATION**

**OTHER RELATED DISEASES**
  **CANCER OF STOMACH AND**
    **ESOPHAGUS**
  **ARTERIOSCLEROSIS**
  **CARDIOVASCULAR DISEASES**

# WHY AIR POLLUTION?

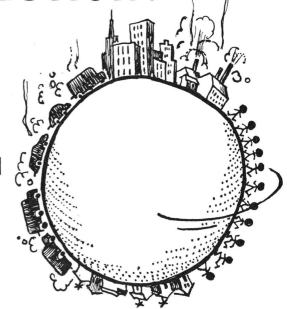

**INCREASED POPULATION**

**EXPANDING INDUSTRY**

**POWER GENERATION FACTORS**

**INCREASED NUMBER OF HOMES**

**NUMBER OF AUTOMOBILES**

**WEATHER AND TEMPERATURE CONDITIONS**

# TYPES OF HEALTH AGENCIES

**Official (Governmental)**

**Voluntary**

**Professional**

**Foundations**

**Youth Groups**

**Commercial**

**Coordinating**

**Service Clubs**

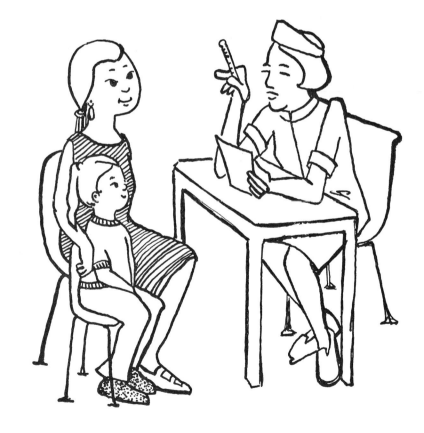

# LEADING CAUSES OF DEATH IN THE UNITED STATES

| CAUSE OF DEATH (TODAY) | 1900 |
|---|:---:|
| 1. CARDIOVASCULAR DISEASE | 4 |
| 2. MALIGNANT NEOPLASMS | 8 |
| 3. VASCULAR LESIONS OF THE CNS | 5 |
| 4. ACCIDENTS | 7 |
| 5. DISEASES OF EARLY INFANCY | 1 |
| 6. INFLUENZA AND PNEUMONIA | 9 |
| 7. GENERAL ARTERIOSCLEROSIS | |
| 8. DIABETES MELLITUS | |
| 9. OTHER CIRCULATORY DISEASES | |
| 10. OTHER BRONCHOPULMONIC DISEASES | |
| 11. CONGENITAL MALFORMATIONS | |
| 12. CIRRHOSIS OF THE LIVER | |
| 13. SUICIDE | |
| 14. NEPHRITIS AND RENAL SCLEROSIS | 6 |
| 15. OTHER HYPERTENSIVE DISEASE | |
| 16. TUBERCULOSIS | 2 |

# LIFE EXPECTANCY

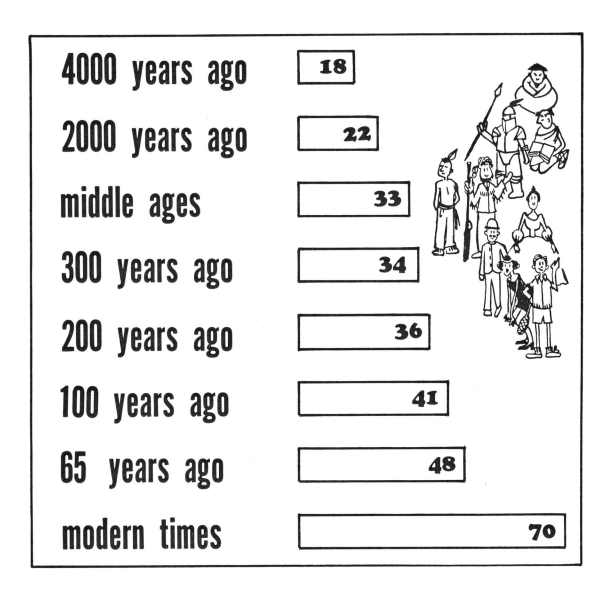

| | |
|---|---|
| 4000 years ago | 18 |
| 2000 years ago | 22 |
| middle ages | 33 |
| 300 years ago | 34 |
| 200 years ago | 36 |
| 100 years ago | 41 |
| 65 years ago | 48 |
| modern times | 70 |